Liu, Xiao

Campbell, Julia

Rethinking Osteoarthritis - Innovative Methods for Sustainable Therapy

A guide for the application of pioneering treatment concepts

bup

Liu, Xiao
Campbell, Julia
Rethinking Osteoarthritis - Innovative Methods for Sustainable Therapy
A guide for the application of pioneering treatment concepts

ISBN: 978-3-69035-858-3

Order number: 2036
Also as an eBook
(978-3-69035-865-1)

Cover design: Kerstin Laube
Production: Michaela Witt

Bremen University Press, 2025.
Fahrenheitstr. 11
28359 Bremen
bup@bremenuniversitypress.com
www.bremenuniversitypress.com

The manuscript may not be used in whole or in part without the prior written consent of the publisher.

This book was printed on environmentally friendly paper from sustainable forestry in order to conserve resources and minimise environmental impact. By using recycled materials and FSC-certified paper, we are helping to protect forests and reduce our ecological footprint.

Disclaimer

This book is for scientific information and general education purposes only. It does not replace individual medical advice, diagnosis or treatment by a licensed physician or other qualified medical professional. Readers should always seek expert medical advice if they have health complaints or questions about the application of the treatment methods described. Some of the treatment methods presented in the book are still undergoing experimental or clinical trials and are not authorised for medical practice in all countries.

Overview

FOREWORD		18
1.	INTRODUCTION	20
2.	PATHOPHYSIOLOGY AND MOLECULAR BASIS OF OSTEOARTHRITIS	25
3.	CLASSIFICATION AND DIAGNOSTIC PROCEDURES	38
4.	CONVENTIONAL TREATMENT METHODS - A CRITICAL APPRAISAL	50
5.	NEW PHARMACOLOGICAL THERAPEUTIC APPROACHES	61
6.	CELL AND MOLECULAR BIOLOGY THERAPIES	80
7.	PHYSICAL AND INSTRUMENTAL METHODS OF ARTHROSIS THERAPY	106
8.	NUTRITION AND MICRONUTRIENT THERAPY	130
9.	PSYCHOLOGICAL AND BEHAVIOURAL THERAPIES	140
10.	INTERDISCIPLINARY AND MULTIMODAL TREATMENT CONCEPTS	149
11.	PERSONALISED MEDICINE AND GENETIC THERAPY APPROACHES	158
12.	THE NEED FOR SURGICAL INTERVENTIONS	176
13.	INTERNATIONAL RESEARCH PERSPECTIVES AND FUTURE DEVELOPMENTS	181
14.	CONCLUDING REMARKS AND CONCLUSION	188
15	TABLE 1: COMPARISON OF CONVENTIONAL AND INNOVATIVE OSTEOARTHRITIS TREATMENTS	191

16	TABLE 2: MOST IMPORTANT MICRONUTRIENTS IN OSTEOARTHRITIS THERAPY	192
17	TABLE 3: OVERVIEW OF REGENERATIVE THERAPIES	193
18	TABLE 4: INFLUENCE OF PSYCHOSOCIAL FACTORS ON THE COURSE OF THE DISEASE	194
19	TABLE 5: COMPARISON OF PHYSICAL THERAPY FORMS	195
20	TABLE 6: OVERVIEW OF DRUG THERAPY OPTIONS FOR OSTEOARTHRITIS	196
21	TABLE 7: CURRENT CLINICAL STUDIES ON INNOVATIVE OSTEOARTHRITIS THERAPIES (SELECTION)	198
22	TABLE 8: PROGNOSTIC FACTORS FOR SUCCESSFUL TREATMENT OF OSTEOARTHRITIS	199
22	TABLE 9: SUMMARY OF THE MOST COMMON BIOMARKERS IN OSTEOARTHRITIS THERAPY	200
23	TABLE 10: PREVENTIVE MEASURES TO AVOID AND DELAY OSTEOARTHRITIS	201
24	TABLE 11: TREATMENT RECOMMENDATIONS ACCORDING TO THE STAGE OF OSTEOARTHRITIS	202
25	TABLE 12: OVERVIEW OF INNOVATIVE THERAPEUTIC PROCEDURES, SUCCESS RATES AND EVIDENCE LEVELS	203
26	COMPLETE BIBLIOGRAPHY	205

Table of contents

FOREWORD 18

1. INTRODUCTION 20
- 1.1 DEFINITION AND DIFFERENTIATION OF OSTEOARTHRITIS 20
- 1.2 HISTORICAL DEVELOPMENT OF OSTEOARTHRITIS TREATMENT 21
- 1.3 EPIDEMIOLOGY AND SOCIO-ECONOMIC SIGNIFICANCE 22
- 1.4 RELEVANCE OF INNOVATIVE TREATMENT METHODS IN THE MEDICAL CONTEXT 23

2. PATHOPHYSIOLOGY AND MOLECULAR BASIS OF OSTEOARTHRITIS 25
- 2.1 ANATOMICAL AND FUNCTIONAL PRINCIPLES OF ARTICULAR CARTILAGE 25
  - 2.1.1 Structure and properties of hyaline cartilage 25
  - 2.1.2 Function of the synovium and joint capsule 26
- 2.2 PATHOPHYSIOLOGICAL CHANGES IN OSTEOARTHRITIS 26
  - 2.2.1 Degeneration of the cartilage tissue 26
  - 2.2.2 Changes in the subchondral bone 27
  - 2.2.3 Formation of osteophytes 27
- 2.3 MOLECULAR MECHANISMS OF CARTILAGE DEGENERATION 28
  - 2.3.1 Imbalance between anabolism and catabolism 28
  - 2.3.2 Role of matrix metalloproteinases (MMP) 28
  - 2.3.3 Apoptosis of chondrocytes 29
- 2.4 ROLE OF INFLAMMATORY MEDIATORS AND CYTOKINES 30
  - 2.4.1 Tumour necrosis factor-α (TNF-α) and interleukin-1β (IL-1β) 30
  - 2.4.2 Involvement of interleukin-6 (IL-6) and interleukin-17 (IL-17) 30
  - 2.4.3 Significance of chronic low-grade inflammation 31
- 2.5 GENETIC AND EPIGENETIC INFLUENCING FACTORS 31
  - 2.5.1 Identification of genetic risk factors 31

	2.5.2	Role of microRNAs and epigenetic regulation	32
2.6		SIGNIFICANCE OF THE SUBCHONDRAL BONE SIGNALS	33
	2.6.1	Vascularisation and angiogenesis in subchondral bone	33
	2.6.2	Mechanotransduction and bone remodelling processes	33
2.7		PAIN MECHANISMS IN OSTEOARTHRITIS	34
	2.7.1	Nociceptive and neuropathic pain components	34
	2.7.2	Central sensitisation and pain chronification	34
	2.7.3	Role of neuroinflammatory processes	35
2.8		BIBLIOGRAPHY (CHAPTERS 1 AND 2)	35
3.		**CLASSIFICATION AND DIAGNOSTIC PROCEDURES**	**38**
3.1		CLASSIFICATION OF OSTEOARTHRITIS ACCORDING TO LOCALISATION AND SEVERITY	38
	3.1.1	Classification according to Kellgren and Lawrence	38
	3.1.2	Clinical relevance of early, middle and late stages	39
3.2		IMAGING PROCEDURES	40
	3.2.1	Conventional X-ray: Indications and limitations	40
	3.2.2	Magnetic resonance imaging: cartilage visualisation and early diagnosis	40
	3.2.3	Computed tomography: analysis of the subchondral structures	41
	3.2.4	Ultrasound: soft tissue diagnostics and joint effusion detection	41
3.3		LABORATORY DIAGNOSTICS AND BIOMARKER RESEARCH	42
	3.3.1	Inflammation markers: CRP, interleukins	42
	3.3.2	Specific cartilage and bone degradation products (COMP, CTX-II)	42
	3.3.3	Future prospects for personalised diagnostics	43
3.4		FUNCTIONAL DIAGNOSTICS AND CLINICAL TESTS	44
	3.4.1	Gait analysis and movement diagnostics	44
	3.4.2	Clinical function tests: WOMAC, Lequesne index	44
	3.4.3	Joint puncture and synovial fluid analysis	45

3.5	USE OF ARTIFICIAL INTELLIGENCE IN DIAGNOSTICS	45
3.5.1	AI-supported image analysis	45
3.5.2	Predictive models for disease progression	46
3.5.3	Opportunities and limitations of digital diagnostics	46
3.6	BIBLIOGRAPHY (CHAPTER 3)	47
4.	**CONVENTIONAL TREATMENT METHODS - A CRITICAL APPRAISAL**	**50**
4.1	PHARMACOLOGICAL THERAPY	50
4.1.1	Non-steroidal anti-inflammatory drugs (NSAIDs): Mechanisms of action and risks	50
4.1.2	Corticosteroid injections: Indications and long-term effects	51
4.1.3	Opioids: use for chronic pain and addiction problems	51
4.1.4	Chondroprotective substances: Glucosamine, chondroitin sulphate - Evidence base	52
4.2	PHYSICAL AND PHYSIOTHERAPEUTIC MEASURES	53
4.2.1	Classical movement therapies	53
4.2.2	Manual therapy and joint mobilisation	54
4.2.3.	Electrotherapy and ultrasound treatments	54
4.2.4	Effect of aquatherapy and controlled stress	54
4.3	SURGICAL INTERVENTIONS	55
4.3.1	Joint endoscopy (arthroscopy): Indication and evidence	55
4.3.2	Osteotomy and joint-preserving operations	55
4.3.3	Arthroplasty: materials, durability and complications	56
4.4	LIMITATIONS AND SIDE EFFECTS OF CONVENTIONAL THERAPIES	57
4.4.1	Insufficient pain control and maintenance of function	57
4.4.2	Drug-induced side effects and complications	57
4.4.3	Economic burdens and supply gaps	58
4.5	BIBLIOGRAPHY (CHAPTER 4)	58

5. NEW PHARMACOLOGICAL THERAPEUTIC APPROACHES 61

5.1 DEVELOPMENT OF SELECTIVE ANTI-INFLAMMATORY AGENTS 61
- 5.1.1 COX-2 inhibitors of the new generation 61
- 5.1.2 Inhibition of specific inflammatory mediators (e.g. IL-1β antagonists) 63

5.2 MODULATION OF SIGNAL PATHS 65
- 5.2.1 Influence on the Wnt/β-catenin signalling pathway 65
- 5.2.2 Inhibition of the TGF-β signalling pathway to reduce fibrosis 66
- 5.2.3 Modulation of the NF-κB signalling pathway to inhibit inflammation 68

5.3 USE OF BIOLOGICS AND MONOCLONAL ANTIBODIES 69
- 5.3.1 IL-6 and IL-17 inhibitors 69
- 5.3.2 Anti-TNF-α therapy: opportunities and limitations 70

5.4 INNOVATIVE PAIN THERAPY 71
- 5.4.1 CGRP antagonists for osteoarthritis-related pain 71
- 5.4.2 Neuromodulators for central pain regulation 72

5.5 EPIGENETIC THERAPY APPROACHES 74
- 5.5.1 Use of histone deacetylase inhibitors 74
- 5.5.2 DNA methylation modulators for gene expression control 76

5.6 BIBLIOGRAPHY (CHAPTER 5) 78

6. CELL AND MOLECULAR BIOLOGY THERAPIES 80

6.1 BASICS OF REGENERATIVE MEDICINE FOR OSTEOARTHRITIS 80
- 6.1.1 Principles of tissue and cell regeneration 80
- 6.1.2 Requirements for biocompatible cell therapies 82

6.2 STEM CELL THERAPY 83
- 6.2.1 Mesenchymal stem cells: Collection, processing and clinical use 83
- 6.2.2 Induced pluripotent stem cells (iPS): potential and risks 85

6.2.3	Allogeneic vs. autologous stem cell therapy	86
6.3	CHONDROCYTE TRANSPLANTS AND TISSUE ENGINEERING	88
6.3.1	Autologous chondrocyte implantation (ACI): first to third generation techniques	88
6.3.2	Development of bioactive scaffolds (scaffolds)	89
6.3.3	3D bioprinting in cartilage regeneration	90
6.4	USE OF EXOSOMES AND MICROVESICLES	90
6.4.1	Biological functions of exosomes in cartilage regeneration	90
6.4.2	Therapeutic potential and current study situation	92
6.5	GENE AND GENE THERAPY	94
6.5.1	Basics of gene modification in osteoarthritis	94
6.5.2	Use of viral vectors for gene transfer	95
6.5.3	CRISPR/Cas9 technology in osteoarthritis research	97
6.6	RISKS AND ETHICAL IMPLICATIONS OF CELLULAR THERAPIES	99
6.6.1	Tumour formation risks with stem cell therapies	99
6.6.2	Immunological reactions and rejection processes	100
6.6.3	Ethical issues in gene therapy	102
6.7	BIBLIOGRAPHY (CHAPTER 6)	104
7.	**PHYSICAL AND INSTRUMENTAL METHODS OF ARTHROSIS THERAPY**	**106**
7.1	BASICS OF PHYSICAL PAIN AND FUNCTIONAL THERAPY	106
7.1.1	Mechanisms of action of physical applications	106
7.1.2	Areas of application and limitations of physical therapy for osteoarthritis	108
7.2	THERMOTHERAPY	110
7.2.1	Heat applications: Indications and effects	110
7.2.2	Cold applications (cryotherapy): Mechanisms of action and areas of application	111
7.3	ELECTROTHERAPY	111
7.3.1	Transcutaneous electrical nerve stimulation (TENS)	111
7.3.2	Medium-frequency and high-frequency therapy	113
7.3.3	Neuromuscular electrical stimulation (NMES)	114

7.4	MAGNETIC FIELD THERAPY	116
7.4.1	Basics of pulsed magnetic field therapy	116
7.4.2	Clinical efficacy and scientific evaluation	117
7.5	ULTRASOUND AND SHOCK WAVE THERAPY	119
7.5.1	Therapeutic ultrasound: forms of application and effects	119
7.5.2	Extracorporeal shock wave therapy (ESWT): Indications and evidence	121
7.6	LASER AND LIGHT THERAPY	123
7.6.1	Low-level laser therapy (LLLT)	123
7.6.2	High-intensity laser therapy (HILT)	125
7.7	COMBINATION THERAPIES AND INTEGRATIVE APPROACHES	126
7.7.1	Multimodal physical therapy programmes	126
7.7.2	Integration into holistic therapy plans	127
7.8	BIBLIOGRAPHY (CHAPTER 7)	127
8.	**NUTRITION AND MICRONUTRIENT THERAPY**	**130**
8.1	INFLUENCE OF NUTRITION ON THE COURSE OF OSTEOARTHRITIS	130
8.1.1	Overweight and mechanical stress on the joints	130
8.1.2	Food components that promote and inhibit inflammation	130
8.2	MICRONUTRIENT THERAPY	132
8.2.1	Vitamin D and calcium in bone metabolism	132
8.2.2	Importance of omega-3 fatty acids for cartilage health	132
8.2.3	Trace elements: Zinc, selenium and manganese	133
8.3	USE OF ANTIOXIDANTS	134
8.3.1	Effect of vitamins C and E on oxidative processes in cartilage	134
8.3.2	Coenzyme Q10 and its role in cell metabolism	134
8.4	PHYTOTHERAPY	135
8.4.1	Curcumin and its anti-inflammatory effects	135
8.4.2	Ginger, boswellia and other plant extracts	136
8.5	FUNCTIONAL NUTRITION AND DIETS	136

	8.5.1	Mediterranean diet as a protective nutritional concept 136
	8.5.2	Low-carb and ketogenic diets in osteoarthritis therapy 137
8.6		BIBLIOGRAPHY (CHAPTER 8) 138

9. PSYCHOLOGICAL AND BEHAVIOURAL THERAPIES....140

9.1		SIGNIFICANCE OF PSYCHOSOCIAL FACTORS IN OSTEOARTHRITIS 140
	9.1.1	Influence of stress, depression and anxiety on the course of the disease 140
	9.1.2	Cognitive distortions and their effects on pain perception 141
9.2		PSYCHOTHERAPEUTIC APPROACHES IN OSTEOARTHRITIS THERAPY 141
	9.2.1	Cognitive behavioural therapy (CBT) 141
	9.2.2	Acceptance and Commitment Therapy (ACT) 142
9.3		RELAXATION TECHNIQUES AND MINDFULNESS TRAINING 143
	9.3.1	Progressive muscle relaxation according to Jacobson .. 143
	9.3.2	Mindfulness and meditation: MBSR programmes 144
	9.3.3	Biofeedback and its use for chronic pain 144
9.4		EDUCATIONAL PROGRAMMES AND SELF-MANAGEMENT 145
	9.4.1	Patient education for pain management 145
	9.4.2	Development of coping strategies and pain competence 146
9.5		BIBLIOGRAPHY (CHAPTER 9) 147

10. INTERDISCIPLINARY AND MULTIMODAL TREATMENT CONCEPTS 149

10.1		NECESSITY OF AN INTEGRATIVE THERAPY APPROACH 149
	10.1.1	Limits of monotherapeutic interventions 149
	10.1.2	Advantages of combined forms of therapy 149
10.2		MODELS OF MULTIMODAL PAIN THERAPY 150
	10.2.1	Design and structure of multimodal programmes 150
	10.2.2	Evidence and success of interdisciplinary approaches . 151

10.3	INTEGRATION OF INNOVATIVE THERAPIES INTO ESTABLISHED TREATMENT CONCEPTS	152
10.3.1	Use of biological and cellular therapies as part of multimodal programmes	152
10.3.2	Combination of classic and innovative therapeutic approaches	153
10.4	CHALLENGES AND PROSPECTS FOR INTEGRATIVE CARE	154
10.4.1	Organisational and economic hurdles	154
10.4.2	Future prospects for interdisciplinary osteoarthritis treatment	155
10.5	BIBLIOGRAPHY (CHAPTER 10)	155

11. PERSONALISED MEDICINE AND GENETIC THERAPY APPROACHES 158

11.1	BASICS OF PERSONALISED OSTEOARTHRITIS THERAPY	158
11.1.1	Significance of genetic predispositions for the risk of disease	158
11.1.2	Biomarkers for therapy customisation and prognosis assessment	160
11.2	GENETIC DIAGNOSTICS AND INDIVIDUAL RISK PROFILES	162
11.2.1	Methods of genome analysis in osteoarthritis research	162
11.2.2	Development of personalised prevention and treatment strategies	164
11.3	GENE THERAPY AND MOLECULAR INTERVENTIONS	167
11.3.1	Possibilities of targeted gene modification (CRISPR/Cas9 and other methods)	167
11.3.2	Use of viral vectors and non-viral carrier systems	169
11.4	ETHICAL IMPLICATIONS OF GENETIC THERAPY APPROACHES	171
11.4.1	Weighing up medical progress and ethical concerns	171
11.4.2	Regulatory framework and social acceptance	172
11.5	BIBLIOGRAPHY (CHAPTER 11)	173

12. THE NEED FOR SURGICAL INTERVENTIONS 176

12.1	THE CURRENT STATUS OF SURGICAL PROCEDURES IN OSTEOARTHRITIS THERAPY	176
12.2	THE STATE OF RESEARCH: CAN NEW THERAPIES REPLACE SURGICAL INTERVENTIONS?	177
12.3	REALISTIC PERSPECTIVES: WILL OPERATIONS BE SUPERFLUOUS IN THE FUTURE?	178
12.4	CONCLUSION: BETWEEN HOPE AND REALISTIC ASSESSMENT	179

13. INTERNATIONAL RESEARCH PERSPECTIVES AND FUTURE DEVELOPMENTS ... 181

13.1	CURRENT GLOBAL RESEARCH INITIATIVES FOR OSTEOARTHRITIS TREATMENT	181
13.2	TECHNOLOGICAL INNOVATIONS AND THEIR RELEVANCE FOR OSTEOARTHRITIS TREATMENT	182
13.2.1.	Artificial intelligence in diagnostics and therapy planning	182
13.2.2	Progress in biomaterial research for cartilage replacement	182
13.3	International clinical trials and their results	183
13.3.1	Comparison of international study results on innovative therapies	183
13.3.2	Development of international guidelines and therapy recommendations	184
13.4	CONCLUSION: INTERNATIONAL PERSPECTIVES FOR IMPROVED OSTEOARTHRITIS THERAPY	185
13.5	BIBLIOGRAPHY (CHAPTER 13)	186

14. CONCLUDING REMARKS AND CONCLUSION ... 188

15 TABLE 1: COMPARISON OF CONVENTIONAL AND INNOVATIVE OSTEOARTHRITIS TREATMENTS ... 191

16 TABLE 2: MOST IMPORTANT MICRONUTRIENTS IN OSTEOARTHRITIS THERAPY ... 192

17	TABLE 3: OVERVIEW OF REGENERATIVE THERAPIES	193
18	TABLE 4: INFLUENCE OF PSYCHOSOCIAL FACTORS ON THE COURSE OF THE DISEASE	194
19	TABLE 5: COMPARISON OF PHYSICAL THERAPY FORMS	195
20	TABLE 6: OVERVIEW OF DRUG THERAPY OPTIONS FOR OSTEOARTHRITIS	196
21	TABLE 7: CURRENT CLINICAL STUDIES ON INNOVATIVE OSTEOARTHRITIS THERAPIES (SELECTION)	198
22	TABLE 8: PROGNOSTIC FACTORS FOR SUCCESSFUL TREATMENT OF OSTEOARTHRITIS	199
22	TABLE 9: SUMMARY OF THE MOST COMMON BIOMARKERS IN OSTEOARTHRITIS THERAPY	200
23	TABLE 10: PREVENTIVE MEASURES TO AVOID AND DELAY OSTEOARTHRITIS	201
24	TABLE 11: TREATMENT RECOMMENDATIONS ACCORDING TO THE STAGE OF OSTEOARTHRITIS	202
25	TABLE 12: OVERVIEW OF INNOVATIVE THERAPEUTIC PROCEDURES, SUCCESS RATES AND EVIDENCE LEVELS	203
26	COMPLETE BIBLIOGRAPHY	205
	1. GENERAL PRINCIPLES OF OSTEOARTHRITIS	205
	2. CLASSICAL DRUG THERAPY	205
	3. PHYSICAL AND APPARATIVE THERAPY	206
	4. NUTRITIONAL AND MICRONUTRIENT THERAPY	206

5. REGENERATIVE AND BIOLOGICAL THERAPY APPROACHES 207
6. PSYCHOLOGICAL AND BEHAVIOURAL THERAPIES 207
7. INTERDISCIPLINARY AND MULTIMODAL THERAPY 208
8 PERSONALISED MEDICINE AND GENETIC THERAPY 208

Notes

- This book has a modular structure so that each chapter can be read independently without necessarily having to refer back to others.
- Processing status: April 2025

The publisher

Foreword

The treatment of osteoarthritis is now at a decisive turning point. For decades, this chronic degenerative joint disease was regarded as an unstoppable companion of ageing, for which there was at best relief of the symptoms, but no effective therapy to influence the course of the disease. Painkillers, exercise therapy and, in advanced cases, surgical joint replacement dominated the therapeutic strategies.

However, the rapid advances in medical research, particularly in the fields of regenerative medicine, molecular biology and personalised therapy, are now opening up completely new perspectives. Innovative procedures such as stem cell therapy, the use of exosomes, the modulation of genetic risk factors and modern multimodal treatment concepts not only enable effective pain relief, but also increasingly aim to regenerate damaged cartilage tissue and sustainably improve joint function.

This book is dedicated to the systematic presentation of these new, promising treatment methods. It is aimed at medical professionals, researchers and interested patients who would like to gain a comprehensive insight into the current and future possibilities of osteoarthritis therapy.

The aim is to convey well-founded scientific knowledge in a generally understandable and at the same time technically precise manner, to realistically categorise the opportunities and limitations of modern therapy options and to provide an outlook on developments in the coming years.

May this book help to raise awareness of osteoarthritis as a treatable disease and strengthen hope for a better quality of life, even for sufferers with severe disease.

1. Introduction

1.1 Definition and differentiation of osteoarthritis

Osteoarthritis is the most common degenerative disease of the joints worldwide and is characterised by a progressive, non-inflammatory breakdown of the joint cartilage, which leads to functional impairment and often also to considerable pain. As the disease progresses, it not only leads to destruction of the cartilage, but also to changes in the neighbouring joint structures, in particular the subchondral bone, the joint capsule and the surrounding muscles and ligaments. These processes are usually irreversible and have a considerable impact on the quality of life of the affected person.

Differentiating osteoarthritis from other degenerative joint diseases is particularly important, as both the therapeutic approaches and the prognosis can vary greatly. While osteoarthritis is primarily caused by biomechanical overload and age-related wear and tear, other diseases, such as rheumatoid arthritis or psoriatic arthropathy, are characterised by autoimmune and systemic inflammatory processes. The differentiation from osteonecrosis, in which impaired blood flow to the bone leads to joint damage, is also essential for the therapeutic approach.

The international classification is based on the guidelines of the World Health Organisation (WHO) and is formally expressed in the current version of the International Classification of Diseases (ICD-11). There, osteoarthritis is summarised under the code FA00-FA19 and further differentiated according to affected joints and degrees of severity.

1.2   Historical development of osteoarthritis treatment

The treatment of osteoarthritis has a long and chequered history that is closely linked to the general development of medicine. Even in ancient times, scholars such as Hippocrates and Galen were concerned with the relief of joint pain. The therapeutic measures of the time were primarily limited to symptomatic treatments, in particular the use of herbal extracts, massages and heat treatments.

These approaches were pursued further in the Middle Ages, although medical knowledge remained stagnant and was overshadowed by mystical-religious ideas. It was only with the advent of scientific medicine in the 19th century that a systematic understanding of arthritic changes began. The development of X-ray equipment enabled imaging diagnostics for the first time, which got to the bottom of pathological changes in the joint.

An important milestone was the introduction of non-steroidal anti-inflammatory drugs in the middle of the 20th century, which enabled effective symptomatic treatment of inflammatory processes and pain. Surgical procedures developed in parallel, initially in the form of joint-preserving osteotomies and later with the introduction of endoprostheses. In the last two decades, there has been a paradigm shift that is increasingly focussing on regenerative and molecular biological therapies.

This change is the result of a deeper understanding of the complex molecular and cellular processes involved in osteoarthritis, which has opened up new therapeutic perspectives. In particular, advances in stem cell research, regenerative medicine and personalised therapy offer promising approaches that go beyond the mere treatment of symptoms and could actually slow down or even partially reverse the progression of the disease.

1.3 Epidemiology and socio-economic significance

Osteoarthritis is one of the most common diseases worldwide. According to current epidemiological surveys, over 500 million people worldwide are affected by this disease. The prevalence is particularly high in industrialised countries, which is closely linked to demographic change and the increase in risk factors such as obesity and lack of exercise.

The age and gender distribution shows that women of postmenopausal age are particularly frequently affected, which is explained by hormonal changes and reduced protection by oestrogen. While the hip and spinal joints are particularly affected in men, women have a higher prevalence of knee and wrist osteoarthritis.

The socio-economic burden of osteoarthritis is considerable. Direct costs arise from medical treatment, hospitalisation and surgical procedures. There are also indirect costs due to incapacity to work, early retirement and loss of productivity. Studies estimate that the annual costs to European healthcare systems are in the double-digit billion range.

In addition to the economic consequences, the disease has a considerable impact on the quality of life of those affected. Chronic pain, limited mobility and the associated loss of social participation often lead to accompanying mental illnesses such as depression and anxiety disorders. Osteoarthritis is therefore not only a physical illness, but also a socio-medical problem that requires an interdisciplinary approach to treatment.

1.4 Relevance of innovative treatment methods in the medical context

In view of the limited effectiveness and sometimes considerable side effects of conventional treatment methods, the call for innovative, causally effective and long-term tolerable treatment methods is becoming ever louder. Conventional therapies, which are largely limited to relieving pain and improving mobility, do not offer a sustainable solution to the progression of the disease.

The demographic development with a continuous increase in older population groups is also leading to a growing number of patients who are multimorbid and are often no longer suitable for invasive surgical procedures.

Innovative treatment methods that target the molecular causes of the disease open up completely new perspectives. These primarily include regenerative procedures such as stem cell and gene therapy, the targeted use of biologics and monoclonal antibodies as well as the use of modern biotechnological implants. Non-invasive methods such as the use of digital health applications, personalised exercise programmes and innovative pain therapies are also helping to improve treatment outcomes.

In light of these developments, interdisciplinary collaboration between orthopaedics, rheumatology, molecular biology, pharmacology, rehabilitation medicine and health economics is becoming increasingly important. Only through a comprehensive understanding of the underlying biological processes and consideration of individual patient needs can a sustainable and effective treatment of osteoarthritis be realised.

2. Pathophysiology and molecular basis of osteoarthritis

2.1 Anatomical and functional principles of articular cartilage

2.1.1 Structure and properties of hyaline cartilage

Hyaline cartilage is the most common form of cartilage tissue in the human body and covers the joint surfaces of all diarthrodial (movable) joints. It is characterised by a smooth, glass-like structure that enables low-friction movement of the joint surfaces.

The extracellular matrix, which makes up over 95 per cent of the cartilage volume, consists mainly of collagen type II, proteoglycans such as aggrecan and a high concentration of water. This matrix is divided into four functionally different layers: the superficial zone, the transition zone, the deeper zone and the calcified zone. Each of these layers has a specific arrangement of collagen fibres and a different concentration of chondrocytes.

The special biomechanical properties of hyaline cartilage, such as its elasticity under pressure and high load-bearing capacity, result from the complex interaction between the collagen fibrils and the highly viscous proteoglycan-rich matrix.

2.1.2 Function of the synovium and joint capsule

The synovial membrane, also known as synovia, lines the joint cavity and produces synovial fluid. This fluid is not only responsible for lubricating the joint surfaces, but is also the only source of nutrients for the avascular chondrocytes.

The joint capsule surrounds the joint and stabilises the joint structure. It consists of a tight outer fibrous apparatus and an inner synovial membrane. The integrity of the joint capsule is crucial for maintaining intra-articular pressure and ensuring the diffusion of nutrients into the cartilage.

2.2 Pathophysiological changes in osteoarthritis

2.2.1 Degeneration of the cartilage tissue

The pathological process usually begins with an imbalance between catabolic and anabolic metabolic processes in the cartilage. The ability of chondrocytes to synthesise new matrix components decreases, while degradation by matrix metalloproteinases and other proteolytic enzymes increases.

Microscopically, the first signs of degeneration are fine cracks and a rough surface of the cartilage. As it progresses, deeper fissures develop, which can extend to the calcified cartilage zone and finally to the subchondral bone.

2.2.2 Changes in the subchondral bone

With the loss of cartilage, the subchondral bone is directly exposed to mechanical stress. This leads to a reactive compaction of the bone, known as subchondral sclerosis.

In addition, subchondral cysts are formed by the accumulation of synovial fluid in weakened areas of bone. These cysts contribute to instability and further destruction of the joint architecture.

2.2.3 Formation of osteophytes

Another characteristic feature of osteoarthritis is the formation of osteophytes, bony outgrowths at the edges of the joint. These develop as a biomechanical compensatory reaction of the body to enlarge the joint surface and distribute the load better.

Although osteophytes can increase the stability of the joint in the short term, they contribute to the restriction of joint mobility in the long term and are often associated with painful irritation of the surrounding soft tissue.

2.3 Molecular mechanisms of cartilage degeneration

2.3.1 Imbalance between anabolism and catabolism

In healthy cartilage, there is a dynamic balance between anabolic (building up) and catabolic (breaking down) processes. This balance is significantly disturbed in osteoarthritis. The anabolic processes, controlled by growth factors such as insulin-like growth factor 1 (IGF-1) and transforming growth factor-beta (TGF-β), are reduced or their signalling pathways are dysregulated.

At the same time, catabolic mechanisms that drive the degradation of the extracellular matrix dominate. These catabolic processes are primarily promoted by proinflammatory cytokines such as interleukin-1β (IL-1β) and tumour necrosis factor-α (TNF-α), which trigger overexpression of matrix metalloproteinases (MMPs) and ADAMTS (A Disintegrin And Metalloproteinase with Thrombospondin Motifs).

2.3.2 Role of matrix metalloproteinases (MMPs)

The matrix metalloproteinases are a family of enzymes that are responsible for the degradation of the extracellular matrix. MMP-1, MMP-3 and MMP-13 in particular play a central role in the pathogenesis of osteoarthritis. MMP-13, also known as collagenase 3, is the most important enzyme in the degradation of collagen type II, the main component of cartilage.

Under physiological conditions, the activity of the MMPs is controlled by tissue inhibitors of metalloproteinases (TIMPs). In osteoarthritis, this balance is disturbed so that catabolic activity predominates and the cartilage matrix is increasingly destroyed.

2.3.3 Apoptosis of chondrocytes

The programmed cell death rate of chondrocytes is significantly increased in osteoarthritis. Apoptosis is triggered by a variety of factors, including oxidative stressors, proinflammatory cytokines and mechanical overload.

The loss of chondrocytes is particularly critical as they are the only cell type in cartilage that is responsible for the maintenance and regeneration of the matrix. With increasing apoptosis of the chondrocytes, matrix homeostasis deteriorates irreversibly, further accelerating the degenerative process.

2.4 Role of inflammatory mediators and cytokines

2.4.1 Tumour necrosis factor-α (TNF-α) and interleukin-1β (IL-1β)

These two cytokines are the main players in the inflammatory cascade of osteoarthritis. TNF-α and IL-1β promote the production of MMPs and at the same time suppress the synthesis of important matrix components such as collagen type II and aggrecan.

Both cytokines also activate the NF-κB signalling pathway, which plays a key role in the regulation of inflammation. Numerous pro-inflammatory genes are activated via this signalling pathway, which further intensify the inflammatory and degradation process.

2.4.2 Involvement of interleukin-6 (IL-6) and interleukin-17 (IL-17)

IL-6 plays a decisive role in mediating systemic inflammatory processes and contributes to the differentiation of T helper cells of the Th17 type, which in turn induce the production of IL-17.

IL-17 is a strongly pro-inflammatory cytokine that has been found to be increased in joint tissue in osteoarthritis. It promotes the formation of MMPs, intensifies the local inflammatory reaction and contributes to the degradation of cartilage.

2.4.3 Significance of chronic low-grade inflammation

Low-grade inflammation" describes a persistent, subclinical inflammatory activity that does not reach the intensity of acute inflammation, but nevertheless continuously contributes to tissue damage.

This form of inflammation is characteristic of osteoarthritis and is maintained by the continuous activation of synovial cells, macrophages and chondrocytes. The continuous release of inflammatory mediators leads to a self-reinforcing degenerative process that affects both the cartilage and the bone substance.

2.5 Genetic and epigenetic influencing factors

2.5.1 Identification of genetic risk factors

Genetic predisposition plays a significant role in the development of osteoarthritis. Numerous genome-wide association studies (GWAS) have identified specific gene variants that are associated with an increased risk of osteoarthritis.

The most significant genetic risk factors include polymorphisms in the COL2A1 gene, which codes for collagen type

II, a main component of the cartilage matrix. Changes in this gene impair the stability and resilience of the cartilage.

Other relevant genes are ACAN, which regulates the synthesis of aggrecan, and MMP13, which is responsible for the expression of matrix-degrading enzymes. In addition, genes that modulate the inflammatory response, such as IL1B and TNFA, play a decisive role in the predisposition to osteoarthritis.

2.5.2 Role of microRNAs and epigenetic regulation

Epigenetic mechanisms regulate gene expression without changes to the DNA sequence. The most important epigenetic modifications include DNA methylation, histone modifications and the activity of non-coding RNAs, in particular microRNAs.

MicroRNAs are short RNA molecules that suppress the translation of certain genes. In osteoarthritis research, microRNA-140 and microRNA-146 are of particular interest. While microRNA-140 has a protective effect on cartilage homeostasis, microRNA-146 is associated with the regulation of inflammatory processes and the inhibition of catabolic enzymes.

Changes in the methylation pattern of the DNA also lead to dysregulation of important genes that are responsible for the synthesis of cartilage components and the control of inflammatory reactions. These epigenetic changes are potentially reversible, which makes them a promising therapeutic target.

2.6 Significance of the subchondral bone signals

2.6.1 Vascularisation and angiogenesis in subchondral bone

The subchondral bone undergoes profound structural and functional changes during the course of osteoarthritis. Angiogenesis, i.e. the formation of new blood vessels, plays a central role in this process.

These neovascularised areas often penetrate the degenerating cartilage tissue and contribute not only to increased inflammation but also to pathological pain sensitivity. Parallel to angiogenesis, neoinnervation occurs, i.e. the formation of new nerve fibres, which further intensify the pain mechanism.

2.6.2 Mechanotransduction and bone remodelling processes

Mechanotransduction describes the process by which mechanical stress is converted into biochemical signals that regulate the activity of osteoblasts and osteoclasts.

This finely balanced regulation is disturbed in osteoarthritis. Chronic incorrect loading leads to increased activity of osteoclasts, which promote bone resorption, while at the same time the formation of new osteoblasts is uncoordinated and of inferior quality.

The result is subchondral sclerosis with altered bone architecture, which further damages the articular cartilage as the natural shock-absorbing function of the bone is lost. These changes lead to an abnormal load distribution, which further accelerates cartilage degradation.

2.7 Pain mechanisms in osteoarthritis

2.7.1 Nociceptive and neuropathic pain components

Pain in osteoarthritis is caused by both nociceptive and neuropathic mechanisms. The nociceptive pain results from the direct stimulation of pain receptors by mechanical stress and inflammatory mediators in the synovium and joint capsule.

Neuropathic pain occurs when progressive tissue degradation and angiogenesis cause new nerve fibres to grow into regions that were previously insensitive to pain, such as degenerated cartilage and subchondral bone.

2.7.2 Central sensitisation and pain chronification

Chronic pain leads to a neuroplastic change in the central nervous system, known as central sensitisation.

This condition is characterised by a persistent increase in the excitability of nerve cells in the spinal cord and brain, which leads to an increased sensitivity to pain (hyperalgesia) and a perception of pain in response to non-painful stimuli (allodynia).

Central sensitisation plays a decisive role in the chronification of pain and makes the treatment of osteoarthritis particularly complex, as the pain symptoms can persist even if the structural damage has already been treated.

2.7.3 Role of neuroinflammatory processes

Neuroinflammatory processes are inflammations of the nervous system that are triggered by the activation of microglial cells and astrocytes in the spinal cord and brain.

These cells release pro-inflammatory cytokines, which further increase the excitability of the nerve cells and increase sensitivity to pain.

These mechanisms explain why painkillers that only have a peripheral effect often provide insufficient relief in chronic osteoarthritis. Effective pain therapy must therefore also address central mechanisms of action and have a multimodal focus.

2.8 Bibliography (Chapters 1 and 2)

Altman, R. D., & Gold, G. E. (2007). Atlas of Individual Radiographic Features in Osteoarthritis, Revised. *Osteoarthritis and Cartilage*, 15, A1-A56.
https://doi.org/10.1016/j.joca.2006.11.009

Bijlsma, J. W., Berenbaum, F., & Lafeber, F. P. (2011). Osteoarthritis: An update with relevance for clinical practice. *The Lancet*, 377(9783), 2115-2126.
https://doi.org/10.1016/S0140-6736(11)60243-2

Blagojevic, M., Jinks, C., Jeffery, A., & Jordan, K. P. (2010). Risk factors for onset of osteoarthritis of the knee in older adults: A systematic review and meta-analysis. *Osteoarthritis and Cartilage*, 18(1), 24-33. https://doi.org/10.1016/j.joca.2009.08.010

Berenbaum, F. (2013). Osteoarthritis as an inflammatory disease (osteoarthritis is not osteoarthrosis!). *Osteoarthritis and Cartilage*, 21(1), 16-21. https://doi.org/10.1016/j.joca.2012.11.012

Buckwalter, J. A., & Mankin, H. J. (1998). Articular cartilage: Tissue design and chondrocyte-matrix interactions. *Instructional Course Lectures*, 47, 477-486.

Dieppe, P. A., & Lohmander, L. S. (2005). Pathogenesis and management of pain in osteoarthritis. *The Lancet*, 365(9463), 965-973. https://doi.org/10.1016/S0140-6736(05)71086-2

Felson, D. T., & Neogi, T. (2018). Osteoarthritis: Is it a disease of cartilage or of bone? *Arthritis & Rheumatology*, 70(4), 626-631. https://doi.org/10.1002/art.40423

Glyn-Jones, S., Palmer, A. J., Agricola, R., Price, A. J., Vincent, T. L., Weinans, H., & Carr, A. J. (2015). Osteoarthritis. *The Lancet*, 386(9991), 376-387. https://doi.org/10.1016/S0140-6736(14)60802-3

Goldring, M. B., & Goldring, S. R. (2007). Osteoarthritis. *Journal of Cellular Physiology*, 213(3), 626-634. https://doi.org/10.1002/jcp.21258

Hunter, D. J., & Bierma-Zeinstra, S. (2019). Osteoarthritis. *The Lancet*, 393(10182), 1745-1759. https://doi.org/10.1016/S0140-6736(19)30417-9

Loeser, R. F., Goldring, S. R., Scanzello, C. R., & Goldring, M. B. (2012). Osteoarthritis: A disease of the joint as an organ. *Arthritis & Rheumatism*, 64(6), 1697-1707. https://doi.org/10.1002/art.34453

Lotz, M., Loeser, R. F. (2012). Effects of aging on articular cartilage homeostasis. *Bone*, 51(2), 241-248. https://doi.org/10.1016/j.bone.2012.03.023

Neogi, T. (2013). The epidemiology and impact of pain in osteoarthritis. *Osteoarthritis and Cartilage*, 21(9), 1145-1153. https://doi.org/10.1016/j.joca.2013.03.018

Sandell, L. J., & Aigner, T. (2001). Articular cartilage and changes in arthritis: Cell biology of osteoarthritis. *Arthritis Research*, 3(2), 107-113. https://doi.org/10.1186/ar148

Sharma, L. (2021). Osteoarthritis of the knee. *The New England Journal of Medicine*, 384(1), 51-59. https://doi.org/10.1056/NEJMcp1903768

Vincent, T. L. (2019). Mechanoadaptation and mechanosignalling in osteoarthritis. *Current Opinion in Rheumatology*, 31(1), 80-85. https://doi.org/10.1097/BOR.0000000000000567

Zhu, S., Zhu, J., Zhen, G., Hu, Y., An, S., Li, Y., & Qin, L. (2019). Subchondral bone remodelling in osteoarthritis: New therapeutic targets for halting disease progression. *Bone Research*, 7(1), 1-15. https://doi.org/10.1038/s41413-019-0050-x

3. Classification and diagnostic procedures

3.1 Classification of osteoarthritis according to localisation and severity

3.1.1 Classification according to Kellgren and Lawrence

The Kellgren and Lawrence classification is the most commonly used radiological system worldwide for classifying the severity of osteoarthritis. It was developed in 1957 and is based on the extent of visible degenerative changes in X-ray images of the affected joints.

The system comprises five grades:

- Grade 0: No radiological signs of osteoarthritis.

- Grade 1: Doubtful minor joint space narrowing and possible osteophyte formation.

- Grade 2: Significant osteophytes and possible incipient narrowing of the joint space.

- Grade 3: Moderate joint space narrowing, multiple osteophytes, possible sclerosis of the subchondral bone.

- Grade 4: Severe joint destruction with pronounced joint space narrowing, large osteophytes and sclerosis, deformation of the joint surfaces.

This classification is particularly important for epidemiological studies, as it offers standardised comparisons. However, it does not take into account the clinical symptoms or the functional limitations of the patient.

3.1.2 Clinical relevance of early, middle and late stages

The categorisation into early, middle and late stages has become established in clinical practice, as it enables a differentiated selection of therapeutic measures.

- In the early stages, there are often only minor structural changes in the cartilage, which are not always clinically associated with pain. At this stage, there is the best chance of positively influencing the course of the disease through conservative measures and regenerative therapy approaches.

- In the middle stage, the degenerative changes are already more pronounced. The cartilage layer is significantly reduced and the first osteophytes and subchondral sclerosis can be detected. Patients increasingly report load-dependent pain and restricted movement.

- In the late stage, the joint structure is severely damaged. The joint space is severely narrowed or no longer recognisable, osteophyte formation is pronounced and bone deformation is advanced. This phase is characterised by permanent pain, pain at rest and a considerable restriction of mobility. Surgical intervention is often the only remaining indication.

3.2 Imaging procedures

3.2.1 Conventional X-ray: Indications and limitations

Conventional X-rays are still the standard examination for the initial diagnosis of osteoarthritis. It enables the assessment of joint space narrowing, osteophyte formation, subchondral sclerosis and subchondral cysts.

Its advantages lie in its wide availability, low cost and standardised evaluation. The limitations are that early cartilage damage and soft tissue changes cannot be detected. Particularly in the early stages of osteoarthritis, X-ray images are often still unremarkable, although structural cartilage damage already exists.

3.2.2 Magnetic resonance imaging: cartilage visualisation and early diagnosis

Magnetic resonance imaging (MRI) is the gold standard in the early diagnosis of osteoarthritis, as it can image both the joint structures and the soft tissue in detail.

Modern MRI techniques such as T2 mapping and dGEMRIC technology enable a quantitative assessment of cartilage quality and biochemical composition. This means that the loss of proteoglycans in the cartilage can be detected at an early stage before morphological changes become visible.

MRI is particularly suitable for assessing synovitis, subchondral bone oedema and the integrity of the joint capsule. These findings are prognostically significant as they provide information on the progression of the disease.

3.2.3 Computed tomography: analysis of the subchondral structures

Computed tomography (CT) is primarily used for detailed assessment of the subchondral bone, particularly in the case of complex joint deformities or preoperative planning.

High-resolution CT can be used to precisely visualise the three-dimensional joint architecture. CT arthrography, in which a contrast agent is injected directly into the joint, also enables the precise visualisation of cartilage damage and meniscus injuries, particularly in the knee joint.

3.2.4 Ultrasound: soft tissue diagnostics and joint effusion detection

Ultrasound is a valuable diagnostic tool for assessing soft tissue changes, effusions and synovial inflammation.

Modern high-frequency probes can be used to reliably detect joint effusions, Baker's cysts, synovial thickening and osteophytes. The Power Doppler technique also allows visualisation of synovial vascularisation and thus assessment of inflammatory activity.

A major advantage of ultrasound is the possibility of dynamic examination under functional movements and its use as a guide for intra-articular injections.

3.3 Laboratory diagnostics and biomarker research

3.3.1 Inflammation markers: CRP, interleukins

Although osteoarthritis is primarily considered a degenerative disease, systemic and local inflammatory processes are significant influencing factors in the course of the disease. In laboratory diagnostics, the determination of C-reactive protein (CRP) plays an important role, particularly in differentiating it from inflammatory rheumatic diseases.

Elevated CRP values indicate active inflammatory processes, but the CRP in osteoarthritis is usually only slightly elevated or within the normal range, even in the case of florid synovial inflammation.

In addition, the determination of specific cytokines such as interleukin-1β (IL-1β), interleukin-6 (IL-6) and tumour necrosis factor-α (TNF-α) is becoming increasingly important. These markers are often elevated locally in the synovial tissue and synovial fluid, which allows conclusions to be drawn about the inflammatory activity of the joint.

3.3.2 Specific cartilage and bone degradation products (COMP, CTX-II)

A central goal of modern osteoarthritis research is the establishment of biomarkers that enable early diagnosis, the assessment of disease progression and the evaluation of treatment effects.

Cartilage Oligomeric Matrix Protein (COMP) is an important marker for cartilage degeneration. Elevated COMP levels in the blood correlate with the extent of cartilage degeneration and the progression of the disease.

Another important biomarker is the C-telopeptide of type II collagen (CTX-II), which indicates the degradation of type II collagen in the cartilage. High CTX-II levels in urine or serum indicate an active degenerative process.

Although these biomarkers are still undergoing scientific validation, they could become important tools for personalised osteoarthritis treatment in the near future.

3.3.3 Future prospects for personalised diagnostics

Future diagnostics will increasingly rely on individualised biomarker profiles in order to provide precise information on prognosis and individual treatment response.

In addition to proteins, genetic and epigenetic markers such as microRNAs and metabolite profiles are also used. Linking this data in the sense of a multi-omics analysis (genomics, proteomics, metabolomics) will enable individualised therapy planning that can specifically influence the course of the disease.

3.4 Functional diagnostics and clinical tests

3.4.1 Gait analysis and movement diagnostics

Functional diagnostics play an important role in the assessment of osteoarthritis, as they provide objective data on biomechanical stress and movement patterns.

Instrumental gait analysis uses pressure plates, 3D movement analysis systems and sensor technology to precisely record gait parameters such as stride length, stance phases, asymmetries and joint loads.

Gait analysis is of particular clinical relevance when assessing postoperative functional gain or recognising compensatory incorrect loading.

3.4.2 Clinical functional tests: WOMAC, Lequesne index

The standardised recording of symptoms, functional limitations and quality of life is carried out using validated clinical scores.

The Western Ontario and McMaster Universities Osteoarthritis Index (WOMAC) is the most commonly used international questionnaire to measure pain, joint stiffness and physical function.

The Lequesne Index is another established score that is used specifically to record functional limitations in hip and knee osteoarthritis. These tests are easy to use, reproducible and are used both in routine clinical practice and in scientific studies.

3.4.3 Joint puncture and synovial fluid analysis

The puncture of an affected joint can pursue both diagnostic and therapeutic goals.

Analysing the synovial fluid provides valuable information on the degree of inflammation and the disease mechanism. The following parameters are analysed:

- Cell count and differentiation (to differentiate between infectious and inflammatory processes)
- Viscosity of the synovial fluid
- Crystal detection (for the differential diagnosis of gout or pseudogout)
- Biochemical analysis of inflammation and degradation products

Joint puncture can also be used therapeutically to relieve large effusions or as preparation for intra-articular injections.

3.5 Use of artificial intelligence in diagnostics

3.5.1 AI-supported image analysis

Artificial intelligence (AI) is increasingly revolutionising the radiological diagnosis of osteoarthritis. Deep learning algorithms are used to automatically analyse image data, resulting in greater diagnostic precision and faster analysis.

AI-supported programmes are able to detect even subtle changes in the joint structure that are barely visible to the human observer. They can also produce quantitative analyses of cartilage thickness, joint space and osteophyte formation that are objectively reproducible.

3.5.2 Predictive models for disease progression

A key field of application for AI is the development of predictive models that can make predictions about the individual course of a disease based on large amounts of data and complex statistical procedures.

These models integrate imaging data, clinical parameters, biomarker profiles and genetic information. On this basis, personalised risk analyses can be created that enable early intervention in patients who are particularly at risk.

3.5.3 Opportunities and limitations of digital diagnostics

The integration of AI into medical diagnostics holds enormous opportunities, particularly with regard to improved early diagnostics and the optimisation of personalised therapy decisions.

However, there are also limitations. The quality of AI analyses depends largely on the quality and variety of the underlying data. In addition, ethical questions regarding data security, data protection and responsibility for medical decisions need to be clarified.

The future will require close interaction between man and machine, with AI supporting doctors but not replacing them.

3. Bibliography (Chapter 3)

Altman, R. D., & Gold, G. E. (2007). Atlas of Individual Radiographic Features in Osteoarthritis, Revised. *Osteoarthritis and Cartilage*, 15(Supplement A), A1-A56. https://doi.org/10.1016/j.joca.2006.11.009

Buckland-Wright, C. (2004). Subchondral bone changes in hand and knee osteoarthritis detected by radiography. *Osteoarthritis and Cartilage*, 12(Supplement A), S10-S19. https://doi.org/10.1016/j.joca.2003.10.017

Crema, M. D., Roemer, F. W., & Guermazi, A. (2011). Imaging techniques for osteoarthritis. *Best Practice & Research Clinical Rheumatology*, 24(6), 771-788. https://doi.org/10.1016/j.berh.2010.11.005

Felson, D. T., McLaughlin, S., Goggins, J., et al. (2003). Bone marrow edema and its relation to progression of knee osteoarthritis. *Annals of Internal Medicine*, 139(5_Part_1), 330-336. https://doi.org/10.7326/0003-4819-139-5_Part_1-200309020-00007

Hunter, D. J., & Bierma-Zeinstra, S. (2019). Osteoarthritis. *The Lancet*, 393(10182), 1745-1759. https://doi.org/10.1016/S0140-6736(19)30417-9

Kellgren, J. H., & Lawrence, J. S. (1957). Radiological assessment of osteo-arthrosis. *Annals of the Rheumatic Diseases*, 16(4), 494-502. https://doi.org/10.1136/ard.16.4.494

Knoop, J., van der Leeden, M., van der Esch, M., et al. (2011). Association of lower muscle strength with self-reported knee instability in osteoarthritis of the knee: Results from the Amsterdam Osteoarthritis Cohort. *Arthritis Care & Research*, 63(1), 31-38. https://doi.org/10.1002/acr.20339

Loeser, R. F. (2010). Age-related changes in the musculoskeletal system and the development of osteoarthritis. *Clinics in Geriatric Medicine*, 26(3), 371-386.
https://doi.org/10.1016/j.cger.2010.03.002

McAlindon, T. E., Driban, J. B., Henrotin, Y., et al. (2014). Biomarkers for osteoarthritis: Current status and perspectives for the future. *Annals of the Rheumatic Diseases*, 73(1), 8-14. https://doi.org/10.1136/annrheumdis-2013-203726

Neogi, T. (2013). The epidemiology and impact of pain in osteoarthritis. *Osteoarthritis and Cartilage*, 21(9), 1145-1153. https://doi.org/10.1016/j.joca.2013.03.018

Roemer, F. W., Eckstein, F., Hayashi, D., et al. (2014). The role of imaging in osteoarthritis. *Best Practice & Research Clinical Rheumatology*, 28(1), 31-60.
https://doi.org/10.1016/j.berh.2014.01.001

Schiphof, D., van Middelkoop, M., de Klerk, B. M., et al. (2013). The validity of radiographic definitions for knee osteoarthritis: The influence of clinical characteristics.

Osteoarthritis and Cartilage, 21(8), 1100-1106.
https://doi.org/10.1016/j.joca.2013.05.004

Vincent, T. L., & Watt, F. M. (2014). Osteoarthritis. *Medicine*, 42(4), 187-190.
https://doi.org/10.1016/j.mpmed.2014.01.006

Zhao, X., Shah, D., Gandhi, K., Wei, W., & Dwibedi, N. (2019). Clinical, humanistic, and economic burden of osteo-arthritis among non-institutionalised adults in the United States. *Osteoarthritis and Cartilage*, 27(11), 1618-1626.
https://doi.org/10.1016/j.joca.2019.07.006

4. Conventional treatment methods - a critical appraisal

4.1 Pharmacological therapy

4.1.1 Non-steroidal anti-inflammatory drugs (NSAIDs): Mechanisms of action and risks

NSAIDs are the most commonly used drugs for the symptomatic treatment of osteoarthritis. They work primarily by inhibiting the cyclooxygenase enzymes (COX-1 and COX-2), which suppresses the synthesis of prostaglandins - central mediators of the pain and inflammatory reaction.

While COX-1 mainly regulates physiological functions in the gastrointestinal tract, kidneys and blood clotting, COX-2 is primarily responsible for the inflammatory response.

The selective COX-2 inhibitors (e.g. celecoxib, etoricoxib) were developed to minimise the gastrointestinal side effects of non-selective NSAIDs (e.g. ibuprofen, diclofenac, naproxen). Nevertheless, long-term use remains problematic.

Common side effects are

- Gastrointestinal complaints through to ulcers and bleeding
- Cardiovascular risks, especially with selective COX-2 inhibitors
- Kidney damage and electrolyte disorders

- Increased risk of thromboembolic events

NSAIDs should therefore only be used when clearly indicated, in the lowest possible effective dose and for the shortest possible period of time.

4.1.2 Corticosteroid injections: Indications and long-term effects

Corticosteroids are often injected intra-articularly to relieve acute inflammatory episodes and pain. They have a strong anti-inflammatory effect by inhibiting phospholipase A2 and thus the arachidonic acid cascade.

Typical indications are

- Acute synovial inflammation with effusion formation
- Reactive inflammation due to mechanical overload
- Short-term bridging until other therapies take effect

In the long term, corticosteroid injections should be viewed critically. Studies show that they have a negative effect on the cartilage structure with repeated use and can accelerate the progression of osteoarthritis. The number of injections per joint should therefore be limited to a maximum of three to four per year.

4.1.3 Opioids: use for chronic pain and dependence problems

For severe chronic pain that no longer responds to other measures, weak and strong opioids are used.

The frequently used preparations include

- Weak opioids: tramadol, tilidine
- Strong opioids: oxycodone, morphine, fentanyl

The effect is achieved by binding to µ, ϰ and δ opioid receptors in the central nervous system, which modulates the perception of pain.

Despite their effectiveness in relieving pain, the use of opioids is problematic due to:

- High risk of dependency and abuse
- Development of tolerance and dose increase
- Side effects such as nausea, constipation, dizziness, cognitive impairment and respiratory depression

Opioids should therefore only be used as part of a multimodal pain management programme and under close medical supervision.

4.1.4 Chondroprotective substances: Glucosamine, chondroitin sulphate - evidence base

Glucosamine and chondroitin sulphate are marketed as so-called chondroprotectants. They are intended to support cartilage regeneration and inhibit the breakdown of the extracellular matrix.

However, the evidence on this is contradictory. While some studies show a slight improvement in pain and function, large, methodologically high-quality studies were unable to demonstrate any significant clinical benefit.

Despite their limited efficacy, these substances remain popular due to their favourable side effect profile, especially among patients who wish to avoid long-term drug therapy with NSAIDs.

4.2 Physical and physiotherapeutic measures

4.2.1 Classical movement therapies

Regular exercise is a cornerstone of arthrosis therapy. Targeted training can improve joint function, increase muscle strength and promote joint stability.

Recommended forms of training are

- Endurance training that is easy on the joints (e.g. cycling, swimming)
- Strengthening exercises for joint-stabilising muscles
- Mobilisation exercises to maintain the range of motion

An individual exercise programme adapted to the severity of the osteoarthritis is crucial in order to avoid overloading the joint.

4.2.2 Manual therapy and joint mobilisation

Manual therapy includes targeted mobilisation techniques to improve joint mobility and reduce muscle tension.

Passive mobilisation loosens adhesions in the joint capsule, stimulates the metabolism in the joint and relieves pain. However, these techniques should only be carried out by specially trained therapists.

4.2.3. Electrotherapy and ultrasound applications

Electrotherapeutic procedures such as transcutaneous electrical nerve stimulation (TENS) are used to relieve pain.

The low-frequency current pulses modulate pain conduction in the spinal cord and promote the release of endorphins produced naturally in the body.

Ultrasound therapy is used to promote localised blood circulation and stimulate cell regeneration in damaged tissue. The effectiveness of these procedures is scientifically controversial, but they are still used in practice, particularly as a complementary measure.

4.2.4 Effect of aquatherapy and controlled exercise

Aquatherapy utilises the buoyant forces of water to enable joint-friendly training while relieving the body weight.

The hydrostatic pressure and water temperature also promote blood circulation and reduce muscular tension.

Controlled exercise as part of functional movement therapy is essential to prevent muscular imbalance and further joint deformity.

4.3 Surgical interventions

4.3.1 Arthroscopy (arthroscopy): Indication and evidence

For many years, arthroscopy was a widely used procedure for treating cartilage damage and removing free joint bodies.

However, current guidelines and studies show that the benefits of arthroscopic procedures for degenerative osteoarthritis are limited.

The indication should therefore be made very critically. It is primarily useful for

- Mechanically blocking free joint bodies
- Meniscus lesions with mechanical complaints
- Localised cartilage damage in otherwise healthy joints

4.3.2 Osteotomy and joint-preserving operations

Osteotomies serve to biomechanically relieve the affected joint area by correcting the joint axis.

Typical procedures are

- Valgising or varus repositioning osteotomies for gonarthrosis
- Pelvic osteotomies for incipient coxarthrosis

These procedures are particularly indicated for younger patients with unilateral joint loading in order to delay joint replacement for as long as possible.

4.3.3 Arthroplasty: materials, durability and complications

The implantation of an artificial joint is the last resort in cases of severe osteoarthritis.

Modern endoprostheses are made of highly resilient materials such as titanium alloys, ceramics and highly cross-linked polyethylene. The durability of today's prostheses is between 15 and 20 years for hip and knee endoprostheses, in some cases even longer.

Possible complications include:

- Infections (prosthesis infections)
- Loosening of the prosthesis
- Thromboembolic complications
- Dislocations with hip prostheses

The choice of the optimal implant and the preoperative preparation have a decisive influence on the long-term result.

4.4 Limitations and side effects of conventional therapies

4.4.1 Insufficient pain control and maintenance of function

Despite intensive drug and physical therapy, pain control remains inadequate in many patients. Particularly in the advanced stages of osteoarthritis, it is often not possible to permanently alleviate the pain and restore quality of life.

The mere treatment of symptoms without any influence on disease progression is a major shortcoming of conventional therapeutic approaches.

4.4.2 Drug-induced side effects and complications

Long-term drug therapies are associated with considerable side effects.

Typical problems include:

- Gastrointestinal complications (NSAID gastropathy)
- Increased risk of myocardial infarction and stroke with COX-2 inhibitors
- Kidney damage due to chronic NSAID use
- Opioid dependence and cognitive side effects

These side effects considerably limit the long-term applicability of pharmacological therapy.

4.4.3 Economic burdens and gaps in supply

The treatment costs for conventional therapies are considerable and represent a significant burden for healthcare systems.

Surgical procedures in particular, such as arthroplasty, cause high direct costs, while incapacity to work and early retirement lead to considerable indirect costs.

At the same time, there are considerable gaps in care, particularly in the area of early diagnosis and the widespread use of evidence-based non-drug therapies.

4.5 Bibliography (Chapter 4)

Bjordal, J. M., Johnson, M. I., Lopes-Martins, R. A., et al. (2007). Short-term efficacy of physical interventions in osteoarthritic knee pain. *Osteoarthritis and Cartilage*, 15(9), 957-963. https://doi.org/10.1016/j.joca.2007.02.011

Bannuru, R. R., Osani, M. C., Vaysbrot, E. E., et al. (2019). OARSI guidelines for the non-surgical management of knee, hip, and polyarticular osteoarthritis. *Osteoarthritis and Cartilage*, 27(11), 1578-1589.
https://doi.org/10.1016/j.joca.2019.06.011

Chou, R., Deyo, R., Friedly, J., et al. (2015). Noninvasive treatments for low back pain. *Agency for Healthcare Research and Quality (US)*.

Conaghan, P. G., Dickson, J., & Grant, R. L. (2008). Care and management of osteoarthritis in adults: Summary of

NICE guidance. *BMJ*, 336(7642), 502-503. https://doi.org/10.1136/bmj.39490.608009.AD

Dagenais, S., Haldeman, S., & Wooley, J. R. (2011). Evidence-informed management of chronic low back pain with prescription medications. *The Spine Journal*, 11(8), 739-760. https://doi.org/10.1016/j.spinee.2011.06.002

Hochberg, M. C., Altman, R. D., April, K. T., et al. (2012). American College of Rheumatology 2012 recommendations for the use of nonpharmacologic and pharmacologic therapies in osteoarthritis of the hand, hip, and knee. *Arthritis Care & Research*, 64(4), 465-474. https://doi.org/10.1002/acr.21596

McAlindon, T. E., Bannuru, R. R., Sullivan, M. C., et al. (2014). OARSI guidelines for the non-surgical management of knee osteoarthritis. *Osteoarthritis and Cartilage*, 22(3), 363-388. https://doi.org/10.1016/j.joca.2014.01.003

Mills, K., Hunt, M. A., & Ferber, R. (2013). Biomechanical deviations during level walking associated with knee osteoarthritis: A systematic review and meta-analysis. *Arthritis Care & Research*, 65(10), 1643-1665. https://doi.org/10.1002/acr.22015

Roubille, C., Martel-Pelletier, J., Raynauld, J. P., et al. (2015). New therapeutic targets in osteoarthritis. *Nature Reviews Rheumatology*, 11(11), 639-648. https://doi.org/10.1038/nrrheum.2015.135

Wieland, L. S., Skoetz, N., Pilkington, K., Vempati, R., D'Adamo, C. R., & Berman, B. M. (2017). Yoga treatment for chronic non-specific low back pain. *Cochrane Database of Systematic Reviews*, (1). https://doi.org/10.1002/14651858.CD010671.pub2

Zhang, W., Nuki, G., Moskowitz, R. W., et al. (2010). OARSI recommendations for the management of hip and knee osteoarthritis: Part III: Changes in evidence following systematic cumulative update of research published through January 2009. *Osteoarthritis and Cartilage*, 18(4), 476-499. https://doi.org/10.1016/j.joca.2010.01.013

5. New pharmacological therapeutic approaches

5.1 Development of selective anti-inflammatory agents

5.1.1 COX-2 inhibitors of the new generation

The selective inhibition of the enzyme **cyclooxygenase-2 (COX-2)** represents an important milestone in the symptomatic pharmacotherapy of osteoarthritis. This enzyme plays a central role in the synthesis of proinflammatory prostaglandins, which are significantly involved in the development of pain and inflammatory reactions in the arthritic joint. In contrast to the classic, non-selective **non-steroidal anti-inflammatory drugs (NSAIDs)**, which block both COX-1 and COX-2, COX-2 inhibitors were specifically developed to achieve the most specific inhibition of inflammatory mediators without negatively affecting the protective functions of COX-1, for example in the gastric mucosa or platelet function.

The inhibition of COX-1 by traditional NSAIDs is associated with a number of undesirable side effects, in particular gastrointestinal ulcers, gastrointestinal bleeding and impaired renal function. These side effects represent a considerable therapeutic risk in a mostly elderly patient group, which often has a multimorbid constitution. The selective inhibition of COX-2 addresses this problem by maintaining the analgesic and anti-inflammatory effects while significantly reducing gastrointestinal toxicity.

Modern representatives of this group of drugs include **celecoxib, etoricoxib** and **parecoxib** in particular. In clinical studies, these active ingredients have shown a demonstrably significant reduction in osteoarthritis-related pain and effective control of inflammatory processes in the joint. In addition, direct comparative studies with non-selective NSAIDs have shown a lower incidence of gastrointestinal complications, which makes the use of these preparations particularly attractive in patients with known gastrointestinal diseases or an increased risk of bleeding.

Nevertheless, the use of COX-2 inhibitors is not without its problems. Numerous epidemiological and clinical studies indicate that these substances can increase the risk of serious **cardiovascular complications**. These include, in particular, **myocardial infarctions, strokes** and **thromboembolic events**. The exact pathophysiological mechanisms of these side effects are not yet fully understood, but it is assumed that the inhibition of COX-2 leads to a shift in the prostanoid balance, which normally ensures a balance between prothrombotic and antithrombotic factors.

For this reason, the indication for treatment with COX-2 inhibitors should always be determined with particular care. Especially in patients with known cardiovascular diseases or risk factors such as high blood pressure, hyperlipidaemia or diabetes mellitus, a strict risk-benefit assessment is required. As far as possible, treatment should be limited to the shortest possible period and the lowest effective dose.

Future pharmacological research will focus intensively on the development of further improved COX-2 inhibitors that have an even higher selectivity for the target enzyme and at the same time offer better safety with regard to cardiovascular risks. The aim is to further optimise the therapeutic balance between efficacy and freedom from side effects in order to make the symptomatic treatment of osteoarthritis both safer and more effective.

5.1.2 Inhibition of specific inflammatory mediators (e.g. IL-1β antagonists)

A particularly promising approach in the modern pharmacological treatment of osteoarthritis is the targeted **blockade of specific proinflammatory cytokines,** which play a central role in the pathogenesis and progression of the disease. The focus here is primarily on **interleukin-1β (IL-1β)**, a key factor in the catabolic metabolism of articular cartilage and a decisive mediator of chronic inflammatory processes in the arthritic joint environment.

IL-1β promotes the expression of a large number of catabolic enzymes, including matrix metalloproteinases (especially MMP-13), which significantly accelerate the degradation of the extracellular cartilage matrix. At the same time, IL-1β inhibits the synthesis of cartilage-protective substances and impairs the regenerative capacity of chondrocytes. This dual effect leads to a progression of cartilage degradation and contributes significantly to the degenerative changes that characterise osteoarthritis.

Against this background, targeted IL-1β antagonists such as **anakinra** were developed, which were originally approved for the treatment of inflammatory rheumatic diseases, in particular rheumatoid arthritis. The therapeutic benefits of these substances are now also being intensively researched in the context of osteoarthritis.

Initial clinical studies show that the targeted blockade of IL-1β can not only reduce the production of catabolic enzymes, but also leads to a significant reduction in the inflammatory reaction in the joint. Furthermore, the results indicate that this treatment has a positive effect on pain symptoms and can possibly slow down the progression of the disease.

Despite these promising approaches, the study results to date are not yet sufficient to justify the widespread clinical use of these substances in osteoarthritis. In particular, there is a lack of large, randomised, controlled studies that clearly demonstrate the long-term efficacy and safety of this form of treatment. In addition, the question remains open as to whether blocking individual cytokines in a complex inflammatory network is actually sufficient to have a lasting effect on osteoarthritis progression, or whether a combination therapy that addresses several pathophysiological target structures simultaneously is required.

Future research will therefore focus on further investigating the therapeutic potential of cytokine blockade, defining optimal dosage and application regimes and evaluating possible long-term side effects. At the same time, new active substances will be developed that enable an even more targeted and effective modulation of the inflammatory environment in the joint in order to achieve a causal and personalised therapy for osteoarthritis in the long term.

5.2 Modulation of signal paths

5.2.1 Influence on the Wnt/β-catenin signalling pathway

The **Wnt/β-catenin signalling pathway** is an essential molecular control mechanism that plays a central role in embryonic development as well as in the regulation of cell proliferation, differentiation and tissue homeostasis. In the context of osteoarthritis, this signalling pathway is of particular importance as it significantly influences the processes of cartilage homeostasis and subchondral bone remodelling. Faulty regulation of this signalling pathway can lead to an imbalance between cartilage-degrading and -building processes, which plays a key role in the pathogenesis of osteoarthritis.

Excessive activation of the Wnt/β-catenin signalling pathway promotes the differentiation of osteoblasts and leads to increased new bone formation in the subchondral region. These processes result in **sclerosis of the subchondral bone**, which adversely alters the mechanical properties of the joint and increases the load on the already degenerated cartilage. At the same time, chronic overactivation of this signalling pathway leads to an inhibition of chondrocyte function, which suppresses the synthesis of cartilage-protective matrix components and promotes chondrocyte apoptosis. These processes accelerate **cartilage degeneration** and contribute significantly to progressive joint destruction.

Against this background, pharmacological **modulation of the Wnt/β-catenin signalling pathway** is becoming increasingly important. The targeted use of inhibitors that control the activity of this signalling pathway could offer a double therapeutic benefit: Firstly, the normalisation of pathological bone remodelling in the subchondral region and secondly, the slowing of cartilage degradation by protecting chondrocyte function. Several specific inhibitors are currently in **preclinical and clinical development**, including molecules that act as Wnt antagonists or direct inhibitors of β-catenin activation.

In the future, targeted intervention in this signalling pathway could be a promising component of causal osteoarthritis therapy, particularly in combination with other molecular approaches that address inflammatory processes and degenerative changes in joint tissue.

5.2.2 Inhibition of the TGF-β signalling pathway to reduce fibrosis

The **transforming growth factor-beta (TGF-β)** signalling pathway plays an extremely complex and sometimes contradictory role in the pathogenesis of osteoarthritis. TGF-β is a multifunctional cytokine involved in a variety of cellular processes, including cell proliferation, differentiation, apoptosis and regulation of the extracellular matrix. While moderate activation of this signalling pathway is beneficial for **cartilage regeneration**, chronically elevated activity leads to pathological remodelling processes affecting both the subchondral bone and the synovial membrane.

In advanced osteoarthritis in particular, **excessive TGF-β activity** is associated with the development of **fibrosis processes**. This pathological fibrosis is characterised by an increased deposition of collagen-containing connective tissue, which contributes to a stiffening of the joint tissue, a reduction in joint mobility and an intensification of the inflammatory processes. In the subchondral bone area, this leads to a disturbed tissue architecture, which further promotes pathological bone remodelling. In the synovium, fibrosis can lead to chronic inflammatory irritation, which further impairs joint function.

The targeted **modulation of the TGF-β signalling pathway** therefore represents an innovative approach to interrupt these harmful processes and restore the homeostasis of the joint tissue. The use of TGF-β inhibitors or specific signalling pathway modulators could **inhibit fibrosis formation**, strengthen the regenerative capacity of the joint tissue and thus slow down the progression of osteoarthritis.

Promising results have so far come primarily from **animal models** in which a significant reduction in fibrotic processes and an improvement in joint function have been achieved by inhibiting the TGF-β signalling pathway. However, clinical applications in humans are still pending, as the systemic inhibition of TGF-β can also have potentially undesirable effects on other tissues and organ systems. Future research approaches will therefore focus on the development of locally effective and tissue-specific modulators that enable selective blockade of the TGF-β signalling pathway in the joint without causing systemic side effects.

5.2.3 Modulation of the NF-κB signalling pathway to inhibit inflammation

Nuclear factor kappa B (NF-κB) is a central transcription factor that plays a key role in the regulation of inflammatory processes. It controls the expression of a large number of genes that are responsible for the production of proinflammatory cytokines, chemokines, adhesion molecules and catabolic enzymes. In the context of osteoarthritis pathogenesis, the NF-κB signalling pathway is significantly involved in the maintenance of chronic inflammatory reactions in the joint and contributes significantly to the catabolic remodelling of the joint tissue.

The activation of NF-κB is typically triggered by inflammatory stimuli, mechanical stress or oxidative damage. Following activation, the transcription factor translocates into the cell nucleus, where it stimulates the transcription of numerous proinflammatory genes. This process leads to an increased release of cytokines such as **interleukin-1β (IL-1β)** and **tumour necrosis factor-alpha (TNF-α)** as well as the induction of matrix metalloproteinases, in particular **MMP-13**, which degrade the cartilage matrix.

Inhibiting the NF-κB signalling pathway is therefore a highly attractive therapeutic approach for specifically interrupting the inflammatory cascade and slowing down the degenerative process in the osteoarthritic joint. Current research is focussing primarily on **IκB kinase (IKK) inhibitors**, which prevent the phosphorylation and degradation of the inhibitor IκB. This inhibits the activation of NF-κB and prevents its translocation into the cell nucleus.

The therapeutic benefit of this signalling pathway modulation lies in a significant **reduction in pro-inflammatory mediators, inhibition of MMP expression** and **protection of the cartilage matrix from further degradation.** Initial preclinical studies have already shown that blocking the NF-κB signalling pathway can significantly reduce not only inflammation but also pain symptoms.

In the long term, the targeted modulation of this signalling pathway could contribute to a more effective control of chronic inflammatory processes in arthritic joints and positively influence the course of the disease. The development of tissue-specific NF-κB inhibitors, which preferentially act in the joint tissue without causing systemic side effects, is one of the central focuses of future pharmacological research.

5.3 Use of biologics and monoclonal antibodies

5.3.1 IL-6 and IL-17 inhibitors

Interleukin-6 (IL-6) is a pro-inflammatory cytokine that plays a central role in the pathogenesis of chronic inflammatory processes, including osteoarthritis. By activating signalling pathways such as JAK/STAT, IL-6 contributes to the maintenance of the inflammatory response, the promotion of osteoclast activity and the inhibition of chondrocyte matrix synthesis.

Tocilizumab, a monoclonal antibody against the IL-6 receptor, has already been approved for rheumatoid arthritis and is currently also being intensively investigated in the context of osteoarthritis. Initial studies indicate a reduction in pain intensity and an inhibition of inflammatory activity in the joint, although the long-term effects on cartilage preservation have not yet been sufficiently proven.

Interleukin-17 (IL-17) is another important inflammatory mediator that particularly increases the expression of matrix metalloproteinases in chondrocytes and thus promotes cartilage degradation. Secukinumab, an IL-17 antibody, has already shown positive results in the treatment of psoriatic arthritis. Its use in osteoarthritis is currently being investigated in phase II clinical trials.

5.3.2 Anti-TNF-α therapy: opportunities and limitations

TNF-α is one of the best-studied pro-inflammatory cytokines in the field of chronic joint diseases. The blockade of TNF-α with monoclonal antibodies such as infliximab, adalimumab or etanercept has become established in rheumatology.

Although these active ingredients have been proven to be effective in inflammatory rheumatic diseases, their significance in osteoarthritis has been controversial to date. The reason for this is that osteoarthritis is primarily a degenerative disease in which inflammation plays a secondary role.

Nevertheless, recent studies show that patients with a pronounced inflammatory component (active synovitis) in particular can benefit from TNF-α blockade. However, its use should be strictly individualised and subject to careful risk-benefit assessment.

5.4 Innovative pain therapy

5.4.1 CGRP antagonists for osteoarthritis-related pain

Calcitonin gene-related peptide (CGRP) is a neuropeptide that plays a central role in the mediation of pain and in the development and maintenance of neurogenic inflammatory processes. CGRP is released in particular by sensory neurones and exerts its effect in both the peripheral nervous system and the central nervous system. Its vasodilatory and pro-inflammatory properties make a decisive contribution to the sensitisation of pain receptors and the intensification of pain sensations.

While CGRP antagonists were originally developed for the treatment of **migraine**, more recent scientific findings show that this mechanism of action also has therapeutic potential in the context of **chronic osteoarthritis-related pain**. Osteoarthritis patients often not only suffer from local mechanically induced pain, but also develop **peripheral and central sensitisation** during the course of the disease, in which neurogenic inflammatory processes and increased activity of the nociceptive system play a significant role. CGRP contributes significantly to this pain-intensifying feedback loop.

Modern CGRP antagonists, which include **erenumab, fremanezumab** and **galcanezumab**, specifically block the CGRP receptors or neutralise the peptide itself. This interrupts the transmission of pain signals at the peripheral level and simultaneously modulates central pain processing. This dual mode of action can lead to a significant **reduction in the sensation of pain** and an improvement in the quality of life of patients with chronic osteoarthritis-related pain.

Although these active ingredients are already being used successfully in migraine therapy, clinical studies on their use in osteoarthritis are currently still at the trial stage. However, initial results suggest that CGRP antagonists could also be an effective option for osteoarthritis patients with **treatment-resistant pain**, particularly those who do not respond adequately to conventional pain medication or cannot tolerate it due to side effects.

A key advantage of these substances is their low gastrointestinal and renal toxicity compared to traditional analgesics and the lack of dependence problems associated with opioids. Future research will focus on defining the optimal use of these agents in osteoarthritis, identifying suitable patient groups and generating long-term data on safety and efficacy.

5.4.2 Neuromodulators for central pain regulation

Chronic pain in osteoarthritis is not exclusively caused by peripheral structural changes such as cartilage damage or bone degeneration, but is also increasingly caused by **central nervous mechanisms**. As the disease progresses, **central sensitisation** can develop, in which the perception of pain in the spinal cord and brain is permanently heightened. This maladaptive change in pain processing means that even minor or non-existent peripheral stimuli are perceived as painful.

Neuromodulators that specifically intervene in the neuronal processing of pain stimuli are used to modulate these central pain mechanisms. These primarily include the active ingredients **pregabalin** and **gabapentin**, which were originally developed for the treatment of neuropathic pain, as well as the **serotonin and noradrenaline reuptake inhibitor (SNRI) duloxetine**, which has both an antidepressant and analgesic effect.

Pregabalin and **gabapentin** modulate the **voltage-gated calcium channels of the α2δ type in the spinal cord**. By blocking these channels, the presynaptic release of excitatory neurotransmitters such as glutamate and substance P is reduced. This leads to a reduction in neuronal excitability and an attenuation of nociceptive signalling. These drugs can significantly reduce the intensity of pain, particularly in patients with pronounced neuropathic pain or central sensitisation.

Duloxetine, on the other hand, acts by **strengthening the descending pain-inhibiting pathways** in the central nervous system. By inhibiting the reuptake of serotonin and noradrenaline, the availability of these neurotransmitters in the synaptic cleft is increased, resulting in improved pain inhibition via the corresponding central nervous control circuits. Duloxetine shows a pronounced pain-relieving effect, particularly in patients with emotional pain intensification or comorbid depressive symptoms.

These neuromodulators are particularly suitable for patients in whom classic analgesics are insufficiently effective or contraindicated. These substances represent an important addition to the therapeutic repertoire, particularly in cases of **chronic pain with neuropathic components** or in patients suffering from pronounced **central sensitisation**.

In the long term, further research into the central pain mechanisms is crucial in order to optimise the possible applications of neuromodulators and develop personalised therapy concepts that specifically target the individual pain processing patterns of patients. The combination of pharmacological and non-pharmacological methods, such as cognitive behavioural therapy or neuromodulative methods, will also become increasingly important in this context.

5.5 Epigenetic therapy approaches

5.5.1 Use of histone deacetylase inhibitors

The epigenetic regulation of gene expression is a highly complex biological mechanism that makes it possible to switch certain genes on or off without changing the underlying DNA sequence. **Histone deacetylases (HDACs)**, which are involved in the modification of the chromatin structure, play a central role in this process. By removing acetyl groups from histone proteins, these enzymes cause a compaction of the chromatin structure, which makes the transcription of genes more difficult and suppresses their activity. This mechanism is of particular importance in osteoarthritis, as the function of numerous chondroprotective and anti-inflammatory genes can be restricted by such epigenetic repression.

HDAC inhibitors specifically prevent the removal of acetyl groups from histones, which leads to an "open" chromatin structure and facilitates the transcription of previously suppressed genes. In this way, the expression of genes with anti-inflammatory, antioxidant and cartilage-protective properties can be promoted. In addition, HDAC inhibitors also modulate the activity of transcription factors and regulatory proteins that are directly involved in the pathophysiology of osteoarthritis.

Substances such as **vorinostat** and **trichostatin A** are currently being intensively investigated in preclinical models with regard to their ability to inhibit inflammatory processes in the joint, reduce the activity of catabolic enzymes such as matrix metalloproteinases and promote regenerative processes in cartilage tissue. Initial experimental data show that these substances can stimulate the synthesis of cartilage-protective matrix components, inhibit the apoptosis of chondrocytes and modulate pro-inflammatory signalling pathways such as the NF-$\varkappa$B signalling pathway.

Despite these promising findings, the clinical use of HDAC inhibitors for the treatment of osteoarthritis has not yet been established. Research is currently focussed on developing substances that have a targeted effect on the joint tissue without causing systemic side effects. In particular, the focus is on local application forms and the development of tissue-specific HDAC inhibitors in order to ensure high therapeutic efficacy with minimal toxicity. In the long term, the targeted use of

HDAC inhibitors could become an important building block in personalised, causally oriented osteoarthritis therapy.

5.5.2 DNA methylation modulators for gene expression control

Another promising approach in epigenetic regulation is the targeted **modulation of DNA methylation**, which has a decisive influence on gene expression. The methylation of cytosine bases, in particular at the so-called CpG islands in the promoter regions of genes, leads to a repressive chromatin structure and thus to reduced gene activity. In osteoarthritis, it has been shown that there is both **hypermethylation** of genes that code for chondroprotective and anti-inflammatory factors and **hypomethylation** of genes that activate catabolic and pro-inflammatory processes.

This epigenetic imbalance contributes significantly to the progression of osteoarthritis, as important protective mechanisms of the cartilage tissue are deactivated and harmful degradation processes are intensified. The therapeutic approach is to achieve the reactivation of protective genes through targeted **demethylation** and thus promote regenerative processes in the joint.

Substances such as **5-azacytidine** and related demethylating agents were originally developed in oncology to restore the expression of tumour suppressor genes in malignant cells. In the context of osteoarthritis, experimental models also show that targeted demethylation of promoter regions of chondroprotective genes can support the regeneration of cartilage and promote the synthesis of matrix components such as type II collagen and proteoglycans.

However, the therapeutic use of these substances in the field of osteoarthritis has so far been severely limited, as they have a pronounced **cytotoxic effect** and cause non-specific demethylation even in healthy tissue, which can result in considerable side effects . The use of these active ingredients is therefore currently limited to the treatment of severe oncological diseases.

Current research is pursuing the goal of developing specific modulators that enable **the selective influencing of methylation of disease-relevant genes** in the joint without causing systemic toxicity. Innovative concepts such as the development of targeted DNA methyltransferase inhibitors or the combination with highly specific carrier systems that ensure local release in the joint are being investigated. The combination with other epigenetic modulators is also seen as a promising approach for restoring the disturbed gene expression in the arthritic joint.

In the long term, the precise control of DNA methylation could become an important component of innovative and personalised therapeutic strategies aimed at the sustainable restoration of joint homeostasis and have a significant positive influence on the course of osteoarthritis.

5.6 Bibliography (Chapter 5)

Berenbaum, F. (2013). Targeting cytokines in osteoarthritis: A critical review of the current status and future prospects. *Drugs & Aging*, 30(3), 193-201.
https://doi.org/10.1007/s40266-013-0053-8

Chevalier, X., Eymard, F., & Richette, P. (2013). Biologic agents in osteoarthritis: Hopes and disappointments. *Nature Reviews Rheumatology*, 9(7), 400-410.
https://doi.org/10.1038/nrrheum.2013.44

Cohen, S. P., Vase, L., & Hooten, W. M. (2021). Chronic pain: An update on burden, best practices, and new advances. *The Lancet*, 397(10289), 2082-2097.
https://doi.org/10.1016/S0140-6736(21)00393-7

Felson, D. T. (2020). Osteoarthritis as a disease of mechanics. *Osteoarthritis and Cartilage*, 28(1), 1-9.
https://doi.org/10.1016/j.joca.2019.07.011

Goldring, M. B., & Otero, M. (2011). Inflammation in osteoarthritis. *Current Opinion in Rheumatology*, 23(5), 471-478.
https://doi.org/10.1097/BOR.0b013e328349c2b1

Hunter, D. J., Bierma-Zeinstra, S., & Carr, A. J. (2019). Osteoarthritis. *The Lancet*, 393(10182), 1745-1759.
https://doi.org/10.1016/S0140-6736(19)30417-9

Li, X., Wang, Y., & Wang, K. (2021). Advances in the epigenetic regulation of osteoarthritis. *Bone Research*, 9(1), 1-15.
https://doi.org/10.1038/s41413-021-00149-4

Neogi, T. (2013). The epidemiology and impact of pain in osteoarthritis. *Osteoarthritis and Cartilage*, 21(9), 1145-1153. https://doi.org/10.1016/j.joca.2013.03.018

Robinson, W. H., Lepus, C. M., Wang, Q., et al. (2016). Low-grade inflammation as a key mediator of the pathogenesis of osteoarthritis. *Nature Reviews Rheumatology*, 12(10), 580-592. https://doi.org/10.1038/nrrheum.2016.136

Wang, T., & He, C. (2018). Pro-inflammatory cytokines: The link between obesity and osteoarthritis. *Cytokine & Growth Factor Reviews*, 44, 38-50. https://doi.org/10.1016/j.cytogfr.2018.10.002

Wittenauer, R., Smith, L., & Aden, K. (2013). Background Paper 6.12: Osteoarthritis. *World Health Organisation*.

Zhang, W., Moskowitz, R. W., Nuki, G., et al. (2010). OARSI recommendations for the management of hip and knee osteoarthritis: Part III. *Osteoarthritis and Cartilage*, 18(4), 476-499. https://doi.org/10.1016/j.joca.2010.01.013

6. Cell and molecular biology therapies

6.1 Basics of regenerative medicine for osteoarthritis

6.1.1 Principles of tissue and cell regeneration

Regenerative medicine pursues a fundamentally curative approach that aims to restore the structural and functional integrity of damaged tissue through active regeneration processes rather than merely treating it symptomatically. In the context of osteoarthritis, the therapeutic focus is particularly on reconstructing the hyaline cartilage matrix and restoring the biomechanical and functional properties of the affected joint. The aim is to reverse or at least slow down the degenerative changes in the joint cartilage by specifically influencing cellular and molecular processes.

The basis of these regenerative processes is the ability of specialised cells, in particular mesenchymal stem cells and chondrogenic progenitor cells, to synthesise new functional tissue structures. Not only do the proliferative capacities of these cells play a decisive role here, but also their ability to differentiate into specific cell lines that enable the formation of new functional cartilage tissue. In addition, the targeted activation of intracellular signalling pathways is required, which control processes such as matrix synthesis, cell metabolism and cytokine production. The most important molecular signalling pathways include the TGF-β/Smad signalling pathway, the Wnt/β-catenin signalling pathway and the PI3K/Akt/mTOR signalling pathway, each of which plays an essential role in controlling cell proliferation, differentiation and matrix production.

A central element of tissue and cell regeneration is also the provision of a suitable microstructural and biochemical environment that optimally supports the regenerative processes. This is where bioactive carrier materials, so-called scaffolds, are used, which not only serve as structural support scaffolds for the colonisation and organisation of cells, but also release growth factors in a targeted manner and convey mechanical and biochemical signals. Depending on the therapeutic objective, these carrier materials can be resorbable or permanently implantable and often consist of materials such as collagen, hyaluronic acid, polylactide (PLA) or bioactive ceramics.

Successful regeneration also requires an adequate supply of essential growth factors to the tissue, which are molecular control elements that regulate cell proliferation, differentiation and matrix synthesis. The most important of these factors include transforming growth factor-beta (TGF-β), which significantly influences chondrogenic differentiation, fibroblast growth factor (FGF), which promotes cell proliferation, and vascular endothelial growth factor (VEGF), which supports the formation of blood vessels in the surrounding tissue and thus ensures the necessary supply of nutrients and oxygen. TGF-β in particular plays a prominent role in the control of chondrogenic matrix synthesis by stimulating the expression of collagen type II and aggrecan, the two main components of the cartilage matrix.

6.1.2 Requirements for biocompatible cell therapies

For the successful clinical application of cell-based therapies in the field of cartilage regeneration, the cells used must fulfil particularly high requirements. In addition to a pronounced differentiation potential and a high proliferative capacity, unrestricted biocompatibility is crucial in order to avoid immunological rejection reactions and inflammatory processes in the recipient tissue.

A key criterion is the immunological compatibility of the cells used. Ideally, these should come from autologous sources, i.e. directly from the patient's tissue, in order to completely rule out the risk of immunological complications and transplant rejection. In cases where allogeneic (foreign human) or xenogeneic (animal) cell sources are used, comprehensive immunological safety measures must be taken. These include precise HLA typing and the use of immunomodulators to prevent immunological incompatibility and the associated rejection reactions.

Another key criterion is the ability of the cells to differentiate reliably into chondrogenic cell lines and to form stable, functionally resilient cartilage matrix. In particular, the synthesis of collagen type II and aggrecan is required, as these structural proteins are essential for the biomechanical properties of articular cartilage. At the same time, long-term stability of the regenerated tissue must be ensured without a tendency to degeneration or the formation of tumour-like cell clusters.

Ensuring the mechanical resilience of the newly formed cartilage matrix is also of crucial importance. As articular cartilage is exposed to high mechanical stresses, the regenerated tissue must have the required biomechanical properties in order to remain functional in the long term. This requirement places particularly high demands on the quality of matrix synthesis and the correct spatial organisation of the newly formed extracellular matrix.

Autologous cell sources such as mesenchymal stem cells from bone marrow, fatty tissue or the synovial membrane are therefore ideal. These are characterised by a high differentiation capacity and excellent biocompatibility. Allogeneic cell transplants, on the other hand, require strict immunological monitoring. Xenogeneic cell therapies are currently still largely in the preclinical research stage due to considerable immunological risks and ethical concerns.

6.2 Stem cell therapy

6.2.1 Mesenchymal stem cells: Collection, preparation and clinical use

Mesenchymal stem cells (MSCs) are multipotent adult stem cells that are characterised by their high plasticity and their ability to differentiate into various mesodermal cell lineages. In particular, their chondrogenic, osteogenic and adipogenic differentiation makes them a promising therapeutic tool in regenerative medicine and especially in the treatment of osteoarthritis.

MSCs are obtained from various tissue sources, depending on the desired cell quality and characteristics. They are most frequently obtained from bone marrow, as this source has been well researched for decades. They are harvested by bone marrow aspiration, usually from the iliac crest under sterile conditions. An alternative and increasingly popular method is harvesting from fatty tissue, which is obtained via liposuction. Adipose tissue offers the advantage of a high cell count with relatively simple harvesting. Other relevant tissue sources are the umbilical cord, in particular Wharton's jelly, and the synovial membrane, which has a particularly high affinity for chondrogenic differentiation due to its proximity to the joint.

Once the cells have been isolated, they are prepared in specialised cell culture laboratories. Here, the MSCs are expanded in vitro , i.e. they are multiplied under controlled conditions, whereby strict attention is paid to maintaining their differentiation capacity and vitality. A critical phase is the purification of the cell population in order to remove unwanted cell types and potentially pro-inflammatory cells. Preparation concludes with characterisation of the cells, during which the identity of the MSCs is confirmed using surface markers such as CD73, CD90 and CD105, while haematopoietic markers such as CD34 and CD45 must be negative.

MSCs are mainly used clinically by direct intra-articular injection into the affected joint. The aim of this application is that the stem cells are either directly involved in the regeneration of the cartilage tissue by differentiating into chondrocytes or - which is far more frequently the case - create a regenerative microenvironment through the release of growth factors and cytokines. This so-called paracrine effect causes a modulation of the local inflammatory process, the inhibition of catabolic enzymes and the activation of endogenous regeneration processes.

Although preclinical studies and initial clinical applications show promising results in terms of pain relief and functional improvement, the actual ability of MSCs to regenerate fully functional hyaline cartilage has not yet been conclusively proven. Long-term controlled studies are required to definitively define the therapeutic value of MSCs in osteoarthritis therapy.

6.2.2 Induced pluripotent stem cells (iPS): potential and risks

The discovery of induced pluripotent stem cells (iPS cells) by Shinya Yamanaka in 2006 represented a groundbreaking advance in regenerative medicine. By reprogramming somatic body cells into a pluripotent embryonic state, iPS cells can theoretically differentiate into any cell type of the human body. This property opens up new perspectives for patient-specific tissue regeneration, as functional chondrocytes can be generated from the patient's own cells and used for targeted cartilage regeneration.

The particular advantage of iPS technology lies in the possibility of developing customised cell therapies that are completely immunologically compatible. In contrast to embryonic stem cells, iPS cells are also not subject to any ethical restrictions, as they are obtained without destroying embryos.

At the same time, there are considerable risks associated with the use of iPS cells. One of the most critical aspects is the genetic instability of these cells. Somatic cells are reprogrammed through the targeted expression of certain transcription factors such as Oct4, Sox2, Klf4 and c-Myc. In particular, the use of c-Myc, a known oncogene, carries the risk of inducing uncontrolled cell proliferation, which can result in the formation of tumour tissue, especially teratomas.

Particularly stringent safety tests are therefore required for the clinical use of iPS cells. These include comprehensive genetic stability analyses, tumourigenicity studies and precise control of differentiation protocols to ensure that no undifferentiated or degenerated cells are transplanted. Currently, the use of iPS cells in the treatment of osteoarthritis is still at an experimental stage, although initial preclinical studies have already demonstrated the feasibility and regenerative potential. However, widespread clinical application is not expected until long-term safety has been proven.

6.2.3 Allogeneic vs. autologous stem cell therapy

In regenerative medicine, a distinction is made between autologous and allogeneic stem cell therapies, with both approaches having specific advantages and disadvantages.

Autologous stem cell therapy utilises stem cells obtained from the patient's own body. This method offers the decisive advantage of excellent immunological tolerance, as the transplanted cells are recognised by the immune system as the body's own. This eliminates the need for immunosuppressive therapy, which can be associated with considerable side effects and risks. In addition, the risk of transmission of infectious agents is minimised with autologous cells. However, one disadvantage of this method is the limited availability of stem cells, particularly in older patients or patients with severe underlying diseases, where cell quality may be limited.

Allogeneic stem cell therapy uses cells from healthy donors, which enables standardised cell production of high quality and availability. This method offers the advantage that cells can be prepared under optimal conditions and made available in large quantities for immediate use. However, there is a significant risk of immunological rejection reactions, which requires careful immunological coordination between donor and recipient. In many cases, immunosuppressive measures are also necessary, which increase the risk of infections and other side effects.

Current clinical studies are focussing intensively on the comparison of both therapeutic approaches in order to evaluate the long-term efficacy, safety profiles and practical applicability. Initial results indicate that with careful immunological selection of the donor and targeted modification of the cells, allogeneic stem cell therapy can also be a promising and practicable option for cartilage regeneration. In the future, genetically modified, hypoimmunogenic stem cells could also be used to further minimise the risk of immunological reactions.

6.3 Chondrocyte transplants and tissue engineering

6.3.1 Autologous chondrocyte implantation (ACI): first to third generation techniques

Autologous chondrocyte implantation (ACI) is an established procedure for biological cartilage regeneration that has proved particularly successful in the case of circumscribed cartilage defects.

- **First generation:**
  Here, the patient's own chondrocytes are harvested arthroscopically from a non-loaded joint area, expanded in vitro and then implanted into the defect under a sewn-on periosteal membrane. Although the method showed initial success, it was limited by a high rate of hypertrophy of the transplanted cells and uneven matrix formation.

- **Second generation:**
  This improved technique uses bioresorbable collagen membranes instead of the periosteum, which has reduced hypertrophy issues. The membrane also offers better control of cell distribution and a more stable matrix structure.

- **Third generation (matrix-associated chondrocyte implantation, MACI):**
  Here, the cultivated chondrocytes are introduced into a three-dimensional carrier matrix prior to implantation. This matrix ensures an even distribution

of the cells, improves their differentiation and facilitates integration into the surrounding tissue.

Long-term studies confirm that the third generation of ACI leads to significantly better functional results and that revision rates have been significantly reduced compared to previous techniques.

6.3.2 Development of bioactive scaffolds (scaffolds)

A decisive factor for the success of tissue engineering procedures is the development of suitable carrier materials (scaffolds) that mechanically support the cells, promote tissue regeneration and are biodegradable.

Modern scaffolds consist of natural polymers such as collagen, hyaluronic acid or fibrin as well as synthetic materials such as polylactide (PLA) and polyglycolide (PGA).

In addition, bioactive scaffolds are being developed that are enriched with growth factors and signalling proteins in order to specifically control the differentiation of the implanted cells.

One particularly innovative development is the use of "smart scaffolds", which adapt their physicochemical properties depending on physiological conditions and thus actively support cell proliferation and differentiation.

6.3.3 3D bioprinting in cartilage regeneration

The 3D bioprinting approach enables the production of patient-specific, three-dimensional cartilage structures from living cells and biocompatible materials.

This technology makes it possible to precisely reproduce the natural architecture of articular cartilage and to position cells in an ideal spatial arrangement.

Current research is focussed on developing suitable bioinks that ensure both high cell vitality and the necessary mechanical stability of the cartilage tissue.

Although 3D bioprinting is still in the experimental phase, the first clinical pilot applications are already being carried out, particularly in young patients with focal cartilage damage.

6.4 Use of exosomes and microvesicles

6.4.1 Biological functions of exosomes in cartilage regeneration

Exosomes are nanoscale, membrane-bounded extracellular vesicles with a diameter of around 30 to 150 nanometres that are actively released by almost all cell types. They are formed in the endosomal compartment of the cell by the fusion of multivesicular bodies with the plasma membrane. Due to their small size and specific molecular composition, exosomes play a central role in intercellular communication. They transport a large number of bioactive molecules, including proteins, lipids, messenger ribonucleic acids (mRNA) and regulatory micro-ribonucleic acids (microRNA), which can trigger specific signalling transduction processes in target cells.

In the context of cartilage regeneration, exosomes are becoming increasingly important as they are able to transmit regenerative and protective signals to chondral tissue in a targeted manner. In particular, they can stimulate the proliferation of chondrocytes, i.e. the cartilage-forming cells, and at the same time promote their differentiation into a stable, functional phenotype. In addition, exosomes are able to modulate degenerative processes by inhibiting catabolic enzymes such as matrix metalloproteinases, which promote the degradation of the extracellular cartilage matrix. This protective mechanism contributes significantly to the maintenance of cartilage homeostasis and prevents the progressive degeneration of articular cartilage.

Particular attention is being paid to mesenchymal stem cell exosomes (MSC exosomes), as these have shown a high therapeutic potential in preclinical studies. They not only promote the regeneration of cartilage tissue, but also have an inflammation-modulating effect by significantly reducing the expression of pro-inflammatory cytokines such as tumour necrosis factor-alpha (TNF-α) and interleukin-1β (IL-1β). These cytokines play a key role in the development and progression of inflammatory and degenerative joint diseases. At the same time, MSC exosomes have been shown to increase the activity of anti-inflammatory mediators such as interleukin-10 (IL-10), which contributes to a reduction of the inflammatory environment in the joint space.

In addition, exosomes contain a large number of microRNAs that specifically regulate gene expression in chondrocytes and thus promote the synthesis of structural proteins such as collagen type II and aggrecan, which are essential for the biomechanical stability of articular cartilage. These molecular mechanisms emphasise the complex and important role of exosomes in cartilage regeneration.

6.4.2 Therapeutic potential and current study situation

The use of exosomes as a "cell-free" therapy option represents a promising approach in regenerative medicine and offers a number of significant advantages over conventional stem cell therapies. In contrast to the direct transplantation of living cells, there is a significantly lower immunological risk when using exosomes, as they do not contain any complete cell structures and therefore no MHC complexes (Major Histocompatibility Complex) that could trigger an immune reaction. This eliminates the need for complex immunosuppression regimes, which are often required for cell-based therapies.

Another significant advantage is the virtual elimination of the risk of tumour formation. While stem cell therapies can be associated with potential degeneration of the transplanted cells under certain circumstances, exosomes lack this cellular basis, which completely eliminates the risk of tumour development.

In addition, exosomes enable comparatively simple standardisation and industrial production. Controlled cultivation of mesenchymal stem cells and standardised extraction and purification processes allow exosomes to be produced in reproducible quality and quantity. These properties facilitate the development of therapeutic preparations that meet the regulatory requirements for pharmaceuticals and could enable broad clinical application in the long term.

Several clinical studies are currently being conducted to investigate the therapeutic use of MSC exosomes in the treatment of knee osteoarthritis. These studies are primarily focussing on the intra-articular application of exosomes, i.e. their direct injection into the joint space. Initial results from phase I and phase II studies are promising: patients report a significant reduction in osteoarthritis-related pain, measured using standardised pain scales such as the Visual Analogue Scale (VAS), as well as an improvement in joint function and mobility. Imaging procedures such as magnetic resonance imaging (MRI) also indicate a stabilisation of the cartilage structure.

However, reliable long-term data on actual structural cartilage regeneration is not yet available. In most studies, the observation period is a maximum of six to twelve months, which does not allow a conclusive assessment of the regenerative potential. At present, the use of exosomes therefore remains primarily experimental in nature, and a broader clinical application will probably only be possible once comprehensive long-term studies are available. Current research is therefore focussed on defining the optimal dosage regimes, application frequencies and long-term safety of this promising therapeutic option.

6.5 Gene and gene therapy

6.5.1 Basics of gene modification in osteoarthritis

In modern medicine, gene modification represents an innovative approach to the causal treatment of chronic degenerative diseases, including osteoarthritis. In contrast to symptomatic therapies, which merely alleviate the symptoms or slow down the progression of the disease, gene modification aims to directly influence the molecular mechanisms that cause the disease. At the centre of this therapeutic concept is the targeted modification of disease-relevant genes in order to either prevent pathological processes or reactivate the body's own regenerative capacities.

In current osteoarthritis research, two basic strategies of gene modification are being pursued, which are diametrically opposed in their objectives, but both pursue the goal of restoring the disturbed balance between tissue degradation and tissue formation in cartilage tissue.

The first strategy is gene suppression, in which harmful catabolic signalling pathways are specifically inhibited. This is achieved by blocking genes that are responsible for the degradation of the extracellular cartilage matrix. The central targets include genes that control the expression of matrix metalloproteinases such as MMP-1, MMP-3 and, above all, MMP-13. These enzymes play a decisive role in the degradation of collagen type II and aggrecan, the main components of the cartilage matrix. In addition, genes coding for pro-inflammatory cytokines such as interleukin-1β and tumour necrosis factor-α are targeted, as these inflammatory mediators further intensify the catabolic process and inhibit regeneration.

The second strategy is gene enhancement, which aims to promote anabolic, i.e. anabolic, processes. The focus here is on the overexpression of genes that stimulate the synthesis of collagen type II and aggrecan. Both substances are essential for the mechanical resilience and structural integrity of articular cartilage. In addition, attempts are being made to increase the expression of anti-inflammatory cytokines such as interleukin-10, as these can dampen the inflammatory reaction in the joint and thus create a favourable regeneration environment.

In the long term, these genetic interventions are intended to achieve a structural and functional improvement in the degenerated cartilage tissue, which will not only alleviate the symptoms but also have a lasting effect on the course of the disease.

6.5.2 Use of viral vectors for gene transfer

The successful implementation of genetic therapy concepts requires the efficient, safe and targeted introduction of therapeutic genes into the affected cartilage cells. In biomedical research, viral vectors have established themselves as particularly efficient transport vehicles for this purpose, as viruses naturally have a high ability to introduce genetic material into cells.

Three main classes of viral vectors are used in osteoarthritis research, which differ significantly in terms of their biological properties, their safety profiles and their efficacy.

Adenoviruses are frequently used due to their high transfection efficiency and strong, albeit temporary, gene expression. They are able to infect both quiescent and actively dividing cells, which is particularly advantageous in the case of largely post-mitotic chondrocytes. However, a disadvantage of adenoviruses is the strong immunological reaction they can trigger in the recipient organism, which considerably limits the duration of gene expression and applicability in vivo.

The advantage of lentiviruses is that they stably integrate the therapeutic genetic material into the genome of the target cells. This integration enables long-lasting and stable expression of the desired gene, which is particularly advantageous in chronic diseases such as osteoarthritis. However, this integration capability also harbours the risk of genome instability, as unintentional insertions into critical genome regions can lead to oncogenic transformations or other serious disorders.

Adeno-associated viruses (AAV) are considered to be the safest vector variant, as they only cause very low immunological reactions and their genetic material usually remains episomal, i.e. outside the cell nucleus. This significantly reduces the risk of genomic instability. However, the disadvantage of AAV systems is their limited capacity for genetic material, which means that they can only be used for relatively small genes or regulatory elements.

Despite these promising approaches, the use of viral vectors is still associated with significant risks. In addition to the immunological and genetic dangers already mentioned, there are uncertainties regarding the control of gene expression, the long-term consequences of genetic modification and the possible unintentional activation of cell proliferation, which harbours the risk of tumorous degeneration. Numerous research groups worldwide are therefore working on the development of further improved, targeted and safe vector systems that maximise the therapeutic benefits and minimise the risks.

6.5.3 CRISPR/Cas9 technology in osteoarthritis research

CRISPR/Cas9 technology is currently regarded as one of the most revolutionary methods of molecular genome editing. It enables precise, highly specific and efficient interventions in the genetic material of living cells. The system is based on an original bacterial defence strategy against viruses and has been adapted for medical applications in recent years. It allows the targeted inactivation (knock-out) of disease-promoting genes or the targeted modification and activation (knock-in) of genes that support regenerative processes.

In osteoarthritis research, the application of CRISPR/Cas9 opens up completely new therapeutic perspectives. In particular, work is being done on blocking catabolic signalling pathways through targeted gene inactivation. One example of this is the targeted silencing of the gene that codes for matrix metalloproteinase 13 (MMP-13). MMP-13 is largely responsible for the degradation of collagen type II and plays a central role in the progressive degradation of cartilage in osteoarthritis. By specifically deactivating this gene, the pathological degradation of cartilage should be slowed down or, ideally, stopped completely.

At the same time, the possibility of actively promoting regenerative processes is being researched. Here, research is focussing on the targeted activation of genes that are responsible for the formation of the extracellular matrix and the synthesis of anti-inflammatory factors. CRISPR technology is also being used here to reactivate genes that are inhibited in their function in the degenerative environment of osteoarthritis.

Despite the enormous therapeutic potential, the application of this technology harbours considerable safety and ethical challenges. The greatest concern lies in so-called off-target effects, i.e. unintended changes at genome sites that are not the target of the modification. Such changes can have unpredictable biological consequences, ranging from harmless to serious pathological effects. There are also ethical concerns regarding the permanent alteration of the human genome and the possible passing on of such changes to subsequent generations if germline modification is carried out.

The application of CRISPR/Cas9 technology in the treatment of osteoarthritis is currently still at the preclinical research stage. Initial experimental approaches are being tested in vitro on cell cultures and in animal models to validate the efficacy and safety of these interventions. Clinical application in humans is not yet possible and remains a long-term project for the future. The coming years will show to what extent this technology has the potential to fundamentally change the treatment of osteoarthritis and possibly mark a real breakthrough in the field of regenerative medicine.

6.6 Risks and ethical implications of cellular therapies

6.6.1 Tumour formation risks with stem cell therapies

A central risk in the clinical application of stem cell therapies, which has not yet been fully controlled, is the potential development of tumours. This risk is particularly significant when using pluripotent stem cells, which include both embryonic stem cells and induced pluripotent stem cells (iPS cells). Pluripotent stem cells have the ability to differentiate into almost all cell types of the human body. However, this high level of plasticity also harbours the risk of uncontrolled proliferation and the formation of degenerate cell populations.

The formation of so-called teratomas poses a particular risk. Teratomas are tumours that consist of tissue from different germ layers and develop from undifferentiated or only partially differentiated stem cells. These tumours can contain different tissue structures such as skin, bone, nerve tissue or glands and can be either benign or malignant. There is also a risk of aggressive malignant tumours developing from unstable cell populations, which are difficult to treat and pose a considerable risk to the patient.

In order to minimise these risks, rigorous quality control of the cell preparations used is essential. The complete differentiation of stem cells into the desired cell line prior to application is a decisive safety factor in order to prevent undifferentiated, potentially tumour-forming cells from remaining in the organism. Modern differentiation protocols are used to ensure that the stem cells are converted as completely as possible under standardised laboratory conditions.

In addition to differentiation, genetic stability testing of the cell preparations is of crucial importance. Long-term cultures and genetic modifications can lead to mutations in the genome of the stem cells, which increase the risk of degenerative cell proliferation. Therefore, the cells must be systematically examined for chromosomal aberrations, mutations in oncogenic signalling pathways and the expression of cancer-associated genes prior to therapeutic application. Highly sensitive molecular biology techniques such as quantitative polymerase chain reaction, high-throughput sequencing and specialised arrays for detecting genomic instabilities are used for this purpose.

Only through the consistent implementation of these quality and safety standards can the risk of tumour degeneration in the context of stem cell therapies be reduced to an acceptable level. Nevertheless, the tumour risk remains a critical factor that has so far limited the broad clinical application of these promising therapies.

6.6.2 Immunological reactions and rejection processes

Another significant risk associated with stem cell therapies are immunological reactions, which in the worst case can lead to complete rejection of the transplanted cells. While autologous cell therapies, in which the patient's own cells are removed, processed and re-transplanted, are largely immunologically tolerable, allogeneic cell therapies pose a considerable challenge to the immune system.

In the case of allogeneic transplants, in which cells originate from a foreign donor, the immune system recognises the foreign cell structures as a potential threat. This can lead to a pronounced immune response, which manifests itself in local or systemic inflammatory reactions and massively impairs the therapeutic efficacy of the stem cell treatment. In severe cases, acute rejection can occur, which is associated with considerable complications and a complete loss of the transplanted cells.

Various strategies are used to minimise these risks. One option is immunosuppressive concomitant therapy, in which the patient's immune system is suppressed pharmacologically. However, this strategy has considerable side effects, including an increased susceptibility to infections and an increased risk of tumours, which is why it is not considered the optimal long-term solution.

Current research approaches therefore aim to reduce the immunogenicity of the transplanted cells themselves. One innovative approach is the genetic modification of donor cells in order to change the expression of surface molecules that are crucial for immune recognition. This includes, for example, the targeted inactivation of genes that are responsible for the expression of the major histocompatibility complex (MHC). This is intended to prevent the transplanted cells from being recognised as foreign by the recipient's immune system.

Another promising strategy is the use of so-called "immune-masking" technologies. This involves the targeted modification of cell surfaces so that immunologically relevant structures are masked or shielded by biocompatible materials. These technologies are currently still in the experimental phase, but are showing promising results in preclinical studies, which suggest a reduction in immune reactions and improved cell acceptance.

In the long term, the combination of genetic modifications with specific biotechnologies could mean that allogeneic stem cell therapies can also be used safely and effectively without permanent immunosuppression.

6.6.3 Ethical issues of gene therapy

The rapid advances in gene therapy and gene modification raise a number of profound ethical questions that go far beyond the purely medical-technical level. These concern both the treatment of human dignity and the right to self-determination as well as the question of which interventions in human genetic integrity are socially and morally acceptable.

Germline gene therapy, in which genetic modifications are made to a person's germ cells, is a particularly controversial topic. As such interventions have the potential to permanently alter the genetic make-up of future generations, this form of gene therapy is legally prohibited in most countries. The associated risks and the unpredictability of the long-term consequences currently make it impossible to provide a responsible ethical justification for such measures. There are also fears that germline gene therapy could lead to a social divide in which "optimised" people are deliberately bred, which fundamentally calls into question both social and ethical values.

Somatic gene therapy, which only affects somatic cells and therefore has no effect on the genetic material of subsequent generations, is also fraught with complex ethical issues. In particular, the question arises as to how the relationship between the potential medical benefit and the long-term risks, which have not yet been sufficiently researched, should be assessed. Patients must be in a position to give fully informed and voluntary consent, which is a considerable challenge when dealing with highly complex scientific issues.

Another key ethical concern relates to access to these innovative therapies. Gene therapies are currently associated with very high costs and are only available to a small, financially well-off group of patients. This raises questions about social justice and equal access to medical progress. The danger of a so-called "genetic medicine elite" is not just a theoretical consideration, but a real socio-political challenge.

To ensure ethical standards, the protection of patients' rights is a top priority. This includes transparent information about opportunities, risks and uncertainties as well as full respect for patients' right to self-determination. In addition, effective control and regulation of research and application by independent ethics committees is essential. These committees should ensure that medical and scientific developments in the field of gene therapy are always in line with the fundamental ethical principles of human dignity, justice and non-harm.

In conclusion, it should be noted that although gene therapy opens up enormous therapeutic potential, this can only be utilised responsibly if ethical and social guidelines are consistently observed and continuously developed.

6.7 Bibliography (Chapter 6)

Barry, F., & Murphy, M. (2013). Mesenchymal stem cells in joint disease and repair. *Nature Reviews Rheumatology*, 9(10), 584-594. https://doi.org/10.1038/nrrheum.2013.109

Caplan, A. I., & Correa, D. (2011). The MSC: An injury drugstore. *Cell Stem Cell*, 9(1), 11-15. https://doi.org/10.1016/j.stem.2011.06.008

Chahla, J., Cinque, M. E., Piuzzi, N. S., et al. (2016). A call for standardisation in platelet-rich plasma preparation protocols and composition reporting. *Journal of Bone and Joint Surgery*, 99(20), 1769-1779. https://doi.org/10.2106/JBJS.17.01213

De Bari, C., & Luyten, F. P. (2008). Stem cells in the treatment of osteoarthritis. *Annals of the Rheumatic Diseases*, 67(9), 1115-1119. https://doi.org/10.1136/ard.2008.092999

Kouroupis, D., & Correa, D. (2021). Increased mesenchymal stem cell functional potency for enhanced therapeutic applications. *Frontiers in Cell and Developmental Biology*, 9, 626961. https://doi.org/10.3389/fcell.2021.626961

Liu, X., & Hunter, D. J. (2018). Mesenchymal stem cell therapy for osteoarthritis: Current perspectives. *Clinical*

Interventions in Aging, 13, 1749-1760. https://doi.org/10.2147/CIA.S149337

Mendicino, M., Bailey, A. M., Wonnacott, K., Puri, R. K., & Bauer, S. R. (2014). MSC-based product characterisation for clinical trials: An FDA perspective. *Cell Stem Cell*, 14(2), 141-145. https://doi.org/10.1016/j.stem.2014.01.013

Orozco, L., Munar, A., Soler, R., et al. (2013). Treatment of knee osteoarthritis with autologous mesenchymal stem cells: A pilot study. *Transplantation*, 95(12), 1535-1541. https://doi.org/10.1097/TP.0b013e318291a2da

Pham, P. V., Vu, N. B., & Phan, N. K. (2018). 3D-bioprinting technology in regenerative medicine for cartilage repair. *Frontiers in Cell and Developmental Biology*, 6, 87. https://doi.org/10.3389/fcell.2018.00087

Tao, S. C., & Guo, S. C. (2020). Role of extracellular vesicles in osteoarthritis. *Current Pharmaceutical Design*, 26(5), 507-515. https://doi.org/10.2174/1381612826666200129113133

Toghraie, F. S., Chenari, N., Gholipour, M. A., et al. (2012). Treatment of osteoarthritis with infrapatellar fat pad derived mesenchymal stem cells in rabbit model. *Bio-Medical Materials and Engineering*, 22(2), 63-70. https://doi.org/10.3233/BME-2012-0679

Zhou, Y., & Yu, J. (2021). Exosomes as therapeutic vehicles in osteoarthritis. *Biomaterials Science*, 9(6), 1813-1825. https://doi.org/10.1039/D0BM01993D

7. Physical and instrumental methods of arthrosis therapy

7.1 Basics of physical pain and functional therapy

7.1.1 Mechanisms of action of physical applications

Physical medicine is an integrative branch of conservative arthrosis therapy that is based on the targeted application of natural or technically generated forms of energy. These include thermal stimuli (heat and cold), mechanical effects (e.. through massages, vibrations or shock waves), electrical currents (stimulation current, ultrasound) and electromagnetic fields (e.. magnetic field therapy, high-frequency therapy). The aim of these measures is to activate the physiological regeneration processes in the damaged tissue, alleviate pain, improve mobility and stabilise or restore the general functionality of the affected joint structures.

In the specific context of osteoarthritis, physical applications unfold their effect via several interlinked mechanisms that start at different levels of biological stimulus processing.

A key effect of physical measures is the promotion of localised blood circulation. Heat applications such as mud, hot air or infrared radiation lead to vasodilation of the capillaries, which results in a better supply of oxygen and nutrients to the joint tissue. At the same time, the removal of inflammatory mediators and degradation products is facilitated. This increased microcirculation improves cell metabolism in the affected area and thus favours the body's natural repair mechanisms. Another therapeutically relevant aspect is the influencing of inflammatory processes. Cold applications such as ice packs, cold air or cryotherapy lower the local tissue temperature, reduce the activity of pro-inflammatory enzymes and modulate the release of pro-inflammatory cytokines such as interleukin-1β or TNF-α. At the same time, the expression of anti-inflammatory messenger substances such as interleukin-10 can be stimulated, which helps to stabilise the inflammatory environment in the arthritic joint.

Another essential mechanism of action of physical forms of therapy is the analgesic effect, i.e. pain relief. This is achieved, among other things, by inhibiting the nociceptive transmission of stimuli at the spinal level, for example through transcutaneous electrical nerve stimulation (TENS). In addition, the release of endogenous opioids such as endorphins can be stimulated, which leads to natural pain modulation. Mechanical stimuli such as massage or vibration can also trigger pain inhibition via afferent neuronal pathways through the so-called gate control principle.

Last but not least, physical applications help to promote mobility and joint function. Heat and movement applications have a muscle-relaxing effect and reduce joint stiffness, which improves mobility, especially in the morning or after periods of rest. Joint mechanics are also positively influenced, as targeted mobilisation and stretching stimuli loosen adhesions and improve the viscoelastic properties of the joint. This in turn has favourable effects on joint lubrication through synovial fluid and the load distribution within the joint space.

Overall, this results in a complex interplay of physiological effects that makes physical therapy a valuable component of multimodal osteoarthritis treatment - especially in the early stages of the disease.

7.1.2 Areas of application and limitations of physical therapy for osteoarthritis

Physical therapy is primarily used for osteoarthritis in the early and middle stages of the disease, i.e. in phases in which there is still no massive structural joint damage. The aim of the measures is to slow down the progression of the disease, compensate for functional limitations and reduce or completely avoid the use of pharmacological painkillers. Physical therapy can make a significant contribution to maintaining quality of life and occupational and social participation, particularly in the case of mild to moderate symptoms.

A particularly important area of application is intermittent pain control, for example in the case of intermittent inflammatory irritation within the joint. Targeted cold applications can quickly alleviate acute pain, while thermal stimuli can reduce muscle tension in chronic conditions and thus promote joint mobility. The combination of physical measures with active movement therapy (e.. physiotherapy, occupational therapy) often leads to synergistic effects that go beyond mere symptom control.

Physical therapy also plays an important role in a preventative and rehabilitative context. For patients with joint misalignments, muscular imbalances or an increased risk of arthritis, it can help to normalise the load conditions in the joint and halt degenerative changes at an early stage. After surgical procedures such as arthroscopy or joint-preserving measures, it helps to restore mobility and relieve pain.

Despite this wide range of possible applications, physical therapy also has clear limitations. These are particularly evident in advanced stages of osteoarthritis, in which considerable structural changes to the joint have already occurred. These include joint deformities, pronounced cartilage defects, osteophyte formation and bony remodelling processes with mechanical axial misalignment. In these cases, conservative measures alone are no longer sufficient to permanently maintain joint function or effectively control pain.

The effectiveness of physical measures can also be limited in patients with inflammatory activated osteoarthritis (activated osteoarthritis), especially if there is no adequate concomitant drug therapy. In such cases, physical therapy is primarily used for symptomatic relief and to maintain as much residual function as possible, but not to causally influence the course of the disease.

It should also be noted that not all physical procedures are equally well documented scientifically. While the effectiveness of TENS and cryotherapy, for example, has been largely confirmed in clinical studies, the evidence base for procedures such as magnetic field therapy or shock wave therapy is still incomplete or controversial. The selection of suitable measures should therefore always be evidence-based, customised and embedded in a comprehensive overall therapeutic concept.

7.2 Thermotherapy

7.2.1 Heat applications: Indications and effects

Heat therapy is a classic procedure for muscle relaxation, pain relief and improved circulation.

Applications include:

- Hot air irradiation
- Mud packs
- Infrared irradiation
- Hot baths or hydrotherapy

Heat promotes vasodilation, which improves the local metabolism and the supply of nutrients to the cartilage and joint tissue. At the same time, muscle tension is released, which helps to relieve pain.

The main indications for heat applications are chronic pain and stiffness in late-stage osteoarthritis.

7.2.2 Cold applications (cryotherapy): Mechanisms of action and areas of application

Cryotherapy is used for acute inflammatory conditions. The local application of cold causes vasoconstriction, reduces the metabolism in inflamed tissues and inhibits the release of pro-inflammatory mediators.

Typical forms of application:

- Ice packs
- Cold air therapy
- Cold water baths

Application should be limited to short intervals to avoid frostbite and tissue damage.

Indications are in particular

- Acute pain phases in activated osteoarthritis
- Joint effusions
- Post-operative and post-interventional inflammatory conditions

7.3 Electrotherapy

7.3.1 Transcutaneous electrical nerve stimulation (TENS)

Transcutaneous electrical nerve stimulation (TENS) is an established and non-invasive electrotherapeutic procedure that is primarily used to treat chronic pain conditions, including joint pain caused by osteoarthritis. The method is based on the targeted stimulation of peripheral nerves using electrical impulses that are applied via electrodes attached to the surface of the skin.

The therapeutic effect of TENS is essentially mediated by two physiological mechanisms. Firstly, the transmission of nociceptive stimuli in the spinal cord is blocked according to the **gate control theory**. This theory states that the activation of fast-conducting, non-pain-conducting nerve fibres (A-beta fibres) by the electrical impulses can inhibit the transmission of pain signals via slow-conducting C-fibres in the posterior horn of the spinal cord. This reduces or suppresses the sensation of pain in the central nervous system.

Secondly, TENS therapy leads to the **activation of the body's own pain-modulating systems**. By stimulating certain nerve areas, the release of endogenous opioids, in particular beta-endorphins and enkephalins, is stimulated. These neurochemical messengers have a direct pain-relieving effect by blocking the pain receptors in the central nervous system.

The application is usually carried out using adhesive electrodes, which are placed in the area of the painful joint or along the corresponding nerve pathways. The stimulation parameters such as frequency, pulse duration and intensity are customised to achieve an optimal effect. Depending on the settings, TENS therapy can provide immediate pain relief or contribute to a long-term reduction in pain intensity through regular use.

TENS is the preferred treatment for **chronic osteoarthritis pain**, especially when drug-based pain therapy is not sufficiently effective or causes undesirable side effects. A particular advantage of this method is that patients can use it themselves at home after receiving professional instruction. Patients can thus largely control their pain treatment themselves and significantly improve their quality of life.

7.3.2 Medium-frequency and high-frequency therapy

In addition to TENS therapy, medium-frequency and high-frequency methods are also used in electrotherapeutic pain and movement therapy, each of which pursues different therapeutic objectives.

Medium-frequency therapy, which includes interferential current therapy, uses electrical currents in the frequency range between 1,000 and 10,000 Hertz. By superimposing several medium-frequency currents, therapeutically effective low-frequency oscillations are generated in the target tissue. This effect enables **deeper muscle and tissue stimulation** without excessively irritating the skin receptors. The aim is to relieve muscle tension, improve blood circulation in deeper layers of tissue and promote lymphatic drainage. In addition, moderate pain relief can be achieved, which is particularly beneficial for muscular complaints associated with osteoarthritis.

High-frequency therapy works with frequencies ranging from 10 MHz to several hundred MHz and includes procedures such as short-wave therapy (diathermy). This achieves controlled **deep heating of the tissue**, which leads to improved microcirculation, muscle relaxation and pain relief. The increase in tissue temperature boosts the metabolism and promotes the resorption of inflammatory exudates. In addition, the improved blood circulation supports the removal of inflammatory mediators, which can have a positive effect on chronic inflammatory processes in the arthritic joint.

However, radiofrequency therapy should only be used under professional guidance. Improper use can lead to **overheating of the tissue and thermal damage**, particularly in areas with thin skin or tissue or in the vicinity of metallic implants. Careful selection of patients and precise device settings are therefore crucial in order to safely achieve therapeutic effects and avoid complications.

7.3.3 Neuromuscular electrical stimulation (NMES)

Neuromuscular electrical stimulation (NMES) is a specialised electrotherapy procedure that is used specifically to activate and strengthen muscles. This method is particularly important for osteoarthritis-related muscle weaknesses, as muscular imbalances and inadequate joint stabilisation can have a significant negative impact on the progression of osteoarthritis.

A typical area of application for NMES **is quadriceps atrophy in osteoarthritis of the** knee, i.e. advanced wear and tear of the knee joint. As a result of the pain and the associated relieving posture, affected patients increasingly lose the thigh muscles that are important for stabilising the knee joint. This weakening leads to further destabilisation of the joint, which can accelerate the arthritic process. This is where NMES comes in, using electrical impulses to trigger targeted muscle contractions that correspond to the natural training effect.

It is applied using surface electrodes that are positioned directly over the affected muscle groups. The controlled stimulation of the motor nerves induces rhythmic muscle contractions that **promote muscle building and strength development**. This effect not only helps to improve joint stability, but can also significantly increase functional performance in everyday life.

NMES is often used in **post-operative rehabilitation**, for example after joint replacement surgery or arthroscopic procedures, to support the rapid reconstruction of the muscles.

NMES can also be a valuable therapeutic alternative for patients with severely restricted mobility who are unable to perform active muscle training.

It is important that the application begins under professional guidance to ensure correct positioning of the electrodes, optimum adjustment of the impulse parameters and safe execution. When used regularly, NMES can make a significant contribution to the functional restoration of muscle strength and to slowing down the progression of osteoarthritis.

7.4 Magnetic field therapy

7.4.1 Basics of pulsed magnetic field therapy

Pulsed *electromagnetic* field therapy (PEMF) is a modern advancement of classic magnetic field applications. It specifically utilises low-frequency, pulsating electromagnetic fields to therapeutically influence biological processes in the tissue. Unlike static magnetic fields, which have a constant field strength, pulsed magnetic fields are characterised by their dynamic change in frequency and intensity, which enables a deeper and more variable effect on cellular processes.

The biophysical basis of PEMF is based on the principle that electromagnetic fields induce electrical currents in biological tissues. These **induced ionic currents** primarily influence the activity of voltage-gated ion channels in the cell membranes, which leads to a modulation of intracellular calcium levels and other electrochemical processes. Calcium metabolism plays a central role in the regulation of cell metabolism, proliferation and differentiation of cells, including chondrocytes, which are relevant for cartilage regeneration.

In addition, PEMF improves local **blood flow and microcirculation** in the tissue. These effects contribute to a better supply of oxygen and nutrients to the damaged joint tissue and simultaneously promote the removal of harmful metabolites and inflammatory mediators. This supports the body's own repair mechanisms and creates a favourable micro-ecological environment for regeneration processes.

Another therapeutic approach of PEMF is **to influence gene expression**. Studies have shown that certain frequencies and field strengths of pulsed magnetic field therapy can modulate the activity of genes that are associated with the inhibition of inflammatory processes and the promotion of cartilage regenerative signalling pathways. The expression of anti-inflammatory cytokines such as interleukin-10 can be increased and the production of pro-inflammatory mediators such as interleukin-1β and TNF-α can be inhibited at the same time. The synthesis of extracellular matrix components such as collagen type II and aggrecan is also positively influenced by this form of therapy, which can stabilise the cartilage structure in the long term.

PEMF is usually applied using special applicators or magnetic field mats that are able to generate pulsating magnetic fields in a targeted manner in the area of the affected joints. The frequency ranges are typically between 1 and 100 Hertz, whereby the exact choice of frequency and intensity is individually adapted to the symptoms and the therapeutic goal.

7.4.2 Clinical efficacy and scientific evaluation

The scientific evaluation of magnetic field therapy, especially PEMF, is characterised by a certain heterogeneity. While some clinical studies demonstrate a significant benefit of the method in the treatment of osteoarthritis pain and functional limitations, other studies come to the conclusion that no therapeutic benefit beyond the placebo effect can be determined.

Positive results can be found above all in studies that have investigated PEMF in **osteoarthritis of the knee and hip joint**. In several randomised controlled trials, a moderate but significant reduction in pain intensity and an improvement in joint function were observed. Some studies have also shown accelerated functional recovery in post-operative rehabilitation after arthroplasty using PEMF.

However, it should be critically noted that the studies were often conducted under very different conditions, which makes it difficult to compare the results. The frequencies, field strengths, application durations and treatment protocols used vary considerably, which makes it difficult to clearly assess the clinical effectiveness. In addition, some of the positive studies have methodological weaknesses, such as small case numbers, lack of blinding or insufficient long-term observation.

Overall, PEMF is regarded as **a well-tolerated complementary measure** in conservative osteoarthritis therapy **with few side effects**. It is particularly suitable as part of a multimodal therapy that also includes active exercise therapy, medication and other physical applications. Due to its minimal side effects, PEMF can also be used in patients who are unable to fully benefit from pharmacological therapies due to intolerances or contraindications.

Despite the positive individual case reports and some promising study results, magnetic field therapy should not be seen as a substitute for causal or evidence-based therapy. Its use should always be assessed on an individual basis and only as a complementary measure as part of a comprehensive treatment concept. Future, methodologically high-quality long-term studies are required in order to determine the exact significance of this form of therapy in the context of osteoarthritis treatment based on evidence.

7.5 Ultrasound and shock wave therapy

7.5.1 Therapeutic ultrasound: forms of application and effects

Ultrasound therapy is an established procedure in physical medicine that is based on the targeted use of high-frequency sound waves in the frequency range of 0.8 to 3 MHz. These sound waves are introduced into the tissue via special transducers, where they cause both **mechanical** and **thermal effects**. The sound waves generate micro-vibrations in the tissue, which trigger a variety of biological reactions at the cellular level.

One of the most important physiological effects of ultrasound therapy is the **stimulation of microcirculation**. The mechanical stimulation of the vessel walls and the surrounding connective tissue leads to improved blood circulation in the treated area. This effect promotes the removal of harmful metabolic products and facilitates the supply of oxygen and nutrients to the tissue, which is of particular therapeutic importance in degenerative joint areas with poor circulation.

Another key effect is the **improvement in cell metabolic activity**. The mechanical vibrations and the heat they generate increase enzymatic activity in the treated cells and stimulate mitochondrial energy processes. This activates regeneration and repair mechanisms in the damaged cartilage and connective tissue.

Particularly noteworthy is the **promotion of collagen neosynthesis**, an effect that is crucial for structural stabilisation and the long-term preservation of joint function. Collagen is one of the main components of the extracellular matrix in cartilage and connective tissue. By stimulating fibroblastic cell types, the production of collagen types I and II is stimulated, which can improve tissue stability and resilience in the long term.

Therapeutic ultrasound also **reduces pain by influencing nerve conductivity**. The sound waves modulate the excitability of peripheral nerves and thus have a pain-relieving effect. In addition, the release of pain-modulating neurotransmitters is stimulated, which can lead to an improvement in subjective pain symptoms.

With regard to the forms of application, a distinction is made between two main methods:

- **Continuous ultrasound:** The sound waves are emitted without interruption, which primarily leads to significant tissue warming. These thermal effects are beneficial for chronic pain syndromes and muscular tension, as they improve the elasticity of the connective tissue, have a positive effect on the viscosity of the synovial fluid and promote muscle relaxation.

- **Pulsed ultrasound:** This method emits sound waves at short intervals and primarily creates mechanical micro-massages of the tissue. This effect is particularly indicated for acute irritations and sensitive tissue structures, as the heat development remains limited while the mechanical stimuli promote regeneration and lymphatic drainage.

Ultrasound therapy is the preferred treatment for **chronic joint complaints** and **degenerative changes** such as osteoarthritis. This therapy has established itself as a valuable addition to pain treatment and functional improvement, particularly in the area of the knee joint and small peripheral joints.

7.5.2 Extracorporeal shock wave therapy (ESWT): Indications and evidence

Extracorporeal shock wave therapy (ESWT) is a modern, non-invasive procedure that introduces high-energy, mechanical pressure waves into the diseased tissue in a targeted manner. Originally developed in urology to break up kidney stones, ESWT has now established itself as an integral part of orthopaedic pain therapy and the treatment of degenerative joint diseases.

The therapeutic effect of ESWT is based on the generation of **mechanical stimuli** that cause microtraumas in the treated tissue. These controlled micro-injuries stimulate a **biological healing reaction**. As a result of the treatment, growth factors such as **vascular endothelial growth factor (VEGF)** and **transforming growth factor beta (TGF-β)** are released.

These factors are crucial for angiogenesis, i.e. the formation of new blood vessels, and promote cellular regeneration in the area of the damaged joint tissue.

In addition, the mechanical stimulation improves **local blood circulation**, which increases metabolic activity in the treated tissue and facilitates the removal of inflammatory mediators. This process makes a significant contribution to pain relief and improving the functionality of the joint.

Another important mechanism of action of ESWT is **neuromodulation**. The high-energy pressure waves reduce the activity of pain-conducting nerve fibres, which can lead to an immediate reduction in the sensation of pain. This effect is of particular clinical relevance in chronic pain syndromes.

Indications for ESWT include

- **Early to moderate gonarthrosis (osteoarthritis of the knee joint):** In these stages, ESWT can help to reduce pain and improve joint function before irreversible structural damage occurs.

- **Femoropatellar pain syndrome:** ESWT can provide targeted relief and pain relief in the area of the kneecap.

- **Tendinopathies in connection with arthrotic joint changes:** ESWT is successfully used for tendon irritation and degenerative tendon changes to promote the regeneration of the affected structures.

The **clinical effectiveness of ESWT** has been proven by numerous studies, particularly with regard to significant **pain**

relief and a short-term improvement in joint function. These positive effects can usually be seen after just a few treatment cycles and make a significant contribution to improving quality of life.

However, the **long-term structural improvement of cartilage tissue** has not yet been clearly proven. Although preclinical studies provide evidence of regenerative effects in cartilage, these results have not yet been confirmed beyond doubt in large, methodologically high-quality long-term studies in humans. ESWT should therefore be considered primarily as a symptomatic and functional therapy as part of a comprehensive treatment plan.

7.6   Laser and light therapy

7.6.1   Low-level laser therapy (LLLT)

Low-level laser therapy (LLLT), also known as **cold laser therapy**, is a modern physical medicine procedure that specifically uses light in the wavelength range of **600 to 1000 nanometres**. In contrast to high-power lasers, LLLT uses a low energy density, which means that no significant tissue heating occurs. Instead, the laser light unfolds **biostimulative effects** at cellular level, which initiate a variety of regenerative and anti-inflammatory processes.

The therapeutic benefits of LLLT are based on several well-studied molecular mechanisms. At the centre is the **stimulation of mitochondrial cytochrome C oxidase**, a key enzyme in the respiratory chain. Absorption of the laser light increases the activity of this enzyme, which leads to an increase in intracellular **adenosine triphosphate (ATP) production.** ATP is the most important energy source for cellular repair and regeneration processes. Improved energy availability in the cells particularly supports the metabolic activity of chondrocytes and connective tissue cells, which are essential for maintaining and rebuilding the cartilage structure.

Another key mechanism of action of LLLT is the **inhibition of pro-inflammatory cytokines** such as **tumour necrosis factor-α (TNF-α)** and **interleukin-1β (IL-1β)**. Both messenger substances play a central role in the pathophysiology of osteoarthritis, as they promote inflammatory processes in the joint tissue, disrupt cartilage homeostasis and accelerate the breakdown of the extracellular matrix. By specifically inhibiting these cytokines, LLLT helps to stabilise the joint environment and reduce painful inflammatory processes.

In addition, LLLT **promotes collagen synthesis**, in particular the production of type II collagen, which is of great importance for the structural integrity of articular cartilage. The stimulation of cartilage cells contributes to the **maintenance of cartilage homeostasis** and can counteract degenerative processes, even if a complete regeneration of the damaged cartilage cannot be expected.

Clinical studies have shown that LLLT can provide **moderate pain relief** and a **functional improvement in joint mobility** in osteoarthritis, especially when used regularly. The best results are usually achieved when LLLT is used **in combination with other therapeutic measures** such as exercise therapy, drug-based pain therapy and physical applications. The main advantages of LLLT are that it is well tolerated, pain-free and can be carried out on an outpatient basis or at home.

7.6.2 High-intensity laser therapy (HILT)

High-intensity laser therapy (HILT) is a further development of classic laser therapy which, in contrast to LLLT, works with **significantly higher energy densities and laser power.** This higher energy input achieves much deeper tissue penetration, which enables intensive treatment of deeper structures such as muscles, ligaments, joint capsules and even tissue close to the cartilage.

In addition to the well-known **biostimulatory effect** at cellular level, which also plays a role in low-level laser therapy, HILT also has a pronounced **thermal effect**. The tissue heating leads to local **vasodilation**, i.e. an expansion of the blood vessels, which improves **microcirculation** in the treated tissue. This increase in localised blood flow contributes to a better supply of nutrients and oxygen to the affected areas and facilitates the removal of metabolic waste products and inflammatory mediators.

Another important effect of HILT is **muscle relaxation**, which is achieved by heating deep layers of tissue. This effect can be of great therapeutic benefit, particularly in the case of osteoarthritis-related muscle tension in large joints such as the knee, hip and shoulder.

HILT is primarily used for **chronic pain syndromes** and in **rehabilitation following surgery**. Typical areas of application are patients with chronic joint pain in the context of degenerative diseases that do not respond adequately to conventional measures, as well as post-operative patients who are seeking rapid pain reduction and functional recovery.

The scientific evidence on HILT is still **limited**, which is mainly due to the relatively short availability of this technology and the heterogeneous study designs. While high-quality, randomised studies on long-term efficacy are lacking, numerous patients report **significant short-term pain relief** and a **noticeable improvement in joint function** after just a few treatment sessions. These positive effects are mainly attributed to the rapid influence on pain and inflammatory processes as well as the improvement in local tissue regeneration.

Despite the limited number of studies, HILT is increasingly being used in clinical practice as a complementary measure in multimodal treatment concepts. However, it should be used by experienced specialists, as the high energy density can lead to undesirable side effects such as skin burns or deeper tissue damage if used incorrectly.

7.7 Combination therapies and integrative approaches

7.7.1 Multimodal physical therapy programmes

An isolated physical measure often only has a limited effect in osteoarthritis.

Successful treatment programmes combine various physical therapies, adapted to the individual symptoms and stage of the disease.

For example, a combination of heat applications to relax the muscles, followed by neuromuscular electrical stimulation to strengthen the muscles and finally TENS therapy to relieve pain can achieve a synergistic effect.

Such multimodal programmes are also increasingly being used in inpatient and outpatient rehabilitation.

7.7.2 Integration into holistic therapy plans

Physical and instrumental procedures should always be embedded in a comprehensive treatment concept.

The combination of drug therapies, dietary changes, psychological pain management and targeted exercise therapies offers the best chances of a lasting improvement in quality of life.

The interdisciplinary exchange between orthopaedists, physiotherapists, pain therapists and psychologists is of crucial importance in order to ensure individualised, needs-based and successful long-term therapy.

7.8 Bibliography (Chapter 7)

Ay, S., Evcik, D., & Kavuncu, V. (2010). Effectiveness of pulsed electromagnetic field therapy in knee osteoarthritis: A randomised, controlled trial. *Rheumatology International*, 30(3), 357-363. https://doi.org/10.1007/s00296-009-0983-9

Brosseau, L., Wells, G. A., Brosseau, M., et al. (2012). Low level laser therapy (Classes I, II and III) for treating osteoarthritis. *Cochrane Database of Systematic Reviews*, (12), CD010035. https://doi.org/10.1002/14651858.CD010035

Clijsen, R., Leoni, D., Schneebeli, A., & Barbero, M. (2017). The effect of low-level laser therapy on pain in patients with knee osteoarthritis: A systematic review and meta-analysis. *Clinical Rehabilitation*, 31(5), 596-608. https://doi.org/10.1177/0269215516653814

Dantas, L. O., Salvini, T. F., & McAlindon, T. E. (2021). Knee osteoarthritis: Key treatments and emerging therapies. *BMJ*, 372, n567. https://doi.org/10.1136/bmj.n567

Giggins, O. M., Persson, U. M., & Caulfield, B. M. (2013). Biofeedback in rehabilitation. *Journal of NeuroEngineering and Rehabilitation*, 10(1), 60. https://doi.org/10.1186/1743-0003-10-60

Page, M. J., Green, S., McBain, B., et al. (2016). Electrotherapy modalities for osteoarthritis of the knee. *Cochrane Database of Systematic Reviews*, (6), CD002823. https://doi.org/10.1002/14651858.CD002823

Pieber, K., Marth, R., & Schuhfried, O. (2014). The efficacy of transcutaneous electrical nerve stimulation (TENS) for the treatment of chronic pain: A meta-analysis of randomized controlled trials. *Physical Therapy Reviews*, 19(3), 156-163. https://doi.org/10.1179/1743288X14Y.0000000071

Vavken, P., Arrich, F., Schuhfried, O., & Dorotka, R. (2009). Effectiveness of pulsed electromagnetic field therapy in the management of osteoarthritis of the knee: A meta-analysis of randomised controlled trials. *Osteoarthritis and Cartilage*, 17(3), 321-327. https://doi.org/10.1016/j.joca.2008.08.005

Wang, C., Schmid, C. H., Rones, R., et al. (2010). A randomised trial of tai chi for fibromyalgia. *New England Journal of Medicine*, 363(8), 743-754. https://doi.org/10.1056/NEJMoa0912611

Zeng, C., Li, H., Yang, T., et al. (2015). Effectiveness of extracorporeal shockwave therapy for knee osteoarthritis: A systematic review and meta-analysis. *Journal of Orthopaedic Research*, 33(5), 659-666. https://doi.org/10.1002/jor.22816

8. Nutritional and micronutrient therapy

8.1 Influence of nutrition on the course of osteoarthritis

8.1.1 Overweight and mechanical stress on the joints

Being overweight is one of the most significant risk factors for the development and progression of osteoarthritis. The additional body weight increases the mechanical load on the joints, especially the weight-bearing joints such as the knees, hips and the small vertebral joints of the lumbar spine.

Any reduction in weight has a demonstrably positive effect on the course of the disease. Studies show that a reduction in body weight of just five to ten per cent can lead to a significant reduction in pain and an improvement in joint function.

Furthermore, obesity not only mechanically promotes joint degeneration, but also contributes to disease progression via metabolic pathways. Adipose tissue is a hormonally active organ that produces pro-inflammatory cytokines such as interleukin-6 (IL-6), tumour necrosis factor-α (TNF-α) and leptin, which amplify inflammatory processes systemically.

8.1.2 Food components that promote and inhibit inflammation

Diet can contribute significantly to the modulation of inflammatory processes.

Ingredients that promote inflammation:

- Saturated fatty acids (e.g. from animal fats and convenience products)
- Trans fats (especially in industrially processed foods)
- Refined carbohydrates and sugars that stimulate the release of pro-inflammatory mediators
- Excessive consumption of red meat and processed meat

Anti-inflammatory ingredients:

- Omega-3 fatty acids (EPA and DHA) from oily fish, which inhibit the synthesis of pro-inflammatory eicosanoids
- Antioxidants such as vitamin C, vitamin E and phytochemicals (e.g. flavonoids and carotenoids)
- Polyphenols from green tea, berries, olive oil and dark chocolate
- Curcumin from the turmeric root, which inhibits NF-κB activation

A consistent change in diet to an anti-inflammatory diet can have a positive effect on disease activity and reduce the need for pain medication.

8.2 Micronutrient therapy

8.2.1 Vitamin D and calcium in bone metabolism

Vitamin D plays a central role in calcium metabolism and is essential for bone health. A vitamin D deficiency leads to impaired bone mineralisation, which not only promotes osteoporosis but also the progression of osteoarthritis.

Vitamin D also has an immunomodulatory effect and inhibits the release of pro-inflammatory cytokines. Studies show that a low vitamin D status is associated with an increased prevalence and severity of osteoarthritis.

The combined supplementation of vitamin D and calcium is particularly useful in older patients in order to stabilise the bone structure and slow down the subchondral remodelling processes.

8.2.2 Importance of omega-3 fatty acids for cartilage health

Omega-3 fatty acids have a strong anti-inflammatory effect through the formation of resolvins and protectins.

Competitive inhibition of the arachidonic acid metabolism reduces the production of pro-inflammatory eicosanoids, while at the same time promoting anti-inflammatory mediators.

Numerous studies have shown that regular supplementation of omega-3 fatty acids (especially EPA and DHA) can lead to a significant reduction in osteoarthritis pain and an improvement in joint function.

The recommended dosage is 1.5 to 3 grams per day in the form of fish oil capsules or as part of a diet rich in fish.

8.2.3 Trace elements: Zinc, selenium and manganese

Trace elements play an important role in maintaining the body's antioxidant capacity and the stability of cartilage tissue.

- **Zinc** is a component of numerous enzymes that are involved in cell repair and immune modulation. A zinc deficiency impairs cartilage regeneration and promotes inflammatory processes.

- **Selenium** is an essential cofactor of glutathione peroxidase, one of the most important antioxidant enzyme systems. Selenium deficiency can lead to an increased oxidative load on the chondrocytes.

- **Manganese** is involved in the synthesis of proteoglycans, which are essential for the structural integrity of the cartilage matrix.

Targeted supplementation of these trace elements can help to reduce oxidative stress in the joint and slow down cartilage degradation.

8.3 Use of antioxidants

8.3.1 Effect of vitamins C and E on oxidative processes in cartilage

Vitamin C (ascorbic acid) is a key antioxidant in the human body and plays an essential role in the synthesis of collagen, the main component of the cartilage matrix.

In addition, vitamin C protects the cells from oxidative damage caused by free radicals, which are increasingly produced during inflammatory processes in arthritic joints. Studies show that a sufficient supply of vitamin C can slow down the progression of cartilage degeneration.

Vitamin E (tocopherol) is a fat-soluble antioxidant that protects the lipid membranes of chondrocytes from oxidative stress. By inhibiting lipid peroxidation, vitamin E helps to maintain the integrity of cell membranes and reduce inflammation-related damage.

Clinical studies have shown moderate pain relief and improvement in joint function with vitamin E supplementation, especially in combination with other antioxidant substances.

8.3.2 Coenzyme Q10 and its role in cell metabolism

Coenzyme Q10 (ubiquinone) is an essential element of the mitochondrial respiratory chain and therefore crucial for cellular energy production.

It also acts as a powerful antioxidant that protects the chondrocytes from oxidative damage.

A coenzyme Q10 deficiency leads to reduced energy production in the cartilage cells and to increased susceptibility to oxidative stress.

Supplementation studies show that coenzyme Q10 improves mitochondrial function, reduces the release of pro-inflammatory cytokines and can improve the quality of life in patients with chronic degenerative joint disease.

8.4 Phytotherapy

8.4.1 Curcumin and its anti-inflammatory effects

Curcumin, the main active ingredient in turmeric root (Curcuma longa), is known for its strong anti-inflammatory and antioxidant properties.

Curcumin inhibits the activation of the nuclear factor kappa B (NF-$\varkappa$B), which is significantly involved in the development and maintenance of inflammatory processes.

In addition, curcumin blocks the activity of cyclooxygenase-2 (COX-2) and lipoxygenase, which suppresses the synthesis of pro-inflammatory eicosanoids.

Randomised controlled studies show that curcumin in standardised extract forms can achieve comparable pain-relieving effects to non-steroidal anti-inflammatory drugs - but with a significantly better side-effect profile.

8.4.2 Ginger, boswellia and other plant extracts

Ginger (Zingiber officinale) contains bioactive substances such as gingerols and shogaols, which have an anti-inflammatory and pain-relieving effect. Ginger preparations have proven to be particularly effective in relieving pain and improving mobility in cases of knee osteoarthritis.

Boswellia serrata (frankincense) contains boswellic acids, which have an inhibitory effect on 5-lipoxygenase, a key enzyme in the inflammatory metabolism.

Frankincense extracts have been shown to reduce inflammatory activity and relieve pain in arthritic complaints.

Other promising herbal substances are

- **Green tea polyphenols:** Strong antioxidant and anti-inflammatory by inhibiting the NF-$\varkappa$B signalling pathway.

- **Devil's claw (Harpagophytum procumbens):** Pain-relieving and anti-inflammatory, well tolerated for chronic joint pain.

8.5 Functional nutrition and diets

8.5.1 Mediterranean diet as a protective nutritional concept

The Mediterranean diet is characterised by a high proportion of plant-based foods, olive oil as the main source of fat, moderate fish consumption and a low proportion of red meat.

This diet is rich in omega-3 fatty acids, antioxidants, phytochemicals and fibre.

Numerous studies have shown that the Mediterranean diet reduces systemic inflammatory processes, has a positive effect on metabolic syndrome and helps to alleviate chronic pain.

In patients with osteoarthritis, a significant improvement in quality of life and a reduction in painkiller consumption was achieved by switching to a Mediterranean diet.

8.5.2 Low-carb and ketogenic diets in osteoarthritis therapy

In recent studies, low-carbohydrate diets and ketogenic diets have shown positive effects on chronic inflammatory diseases.

Reducing sugar and refined carbohydrates lowers insulin levels and reduces the release of pro-inflammatory cytokines.

The ketogenic diet, which is characterised by an extremely low carbohydrate intake and a high fat content, promotes the formation of ketone bodies, in particular beta-hydroxybutyrate.

This metabolite has a direct anti-inflammatory effect by inhibiting the activation of the NLRP3 inflammasome, a key factor in the regulation of inflammation.

Although long-term studies on the use of ketogenic diets for osteoarthritis are still pending, initial results indicate that both body weight can be reduced and inflammatory processes in the joint can be inhibited.

8.6 Bibliography (Chapter 8)

Arden, N., & Nevitt, M. C. (2006). Osteoarthritis: Epidemiology. *Best Practice & Research Clinical Rheumatology*, 20(1), 3-25. https://doi.org/10.1016/j.berh.2005.09.007

Baker, K. R., Matthan, N. R., Lichtenstein, A. H., et al. (2011). Association of plasma phospholipid n-3 and n-6 fatty acids with physical function in mobility-limited older adults. *European Journal of Clinical Nutrition*, 65(3), 282-289. https://doi.org/10.1038/ejcn.2010.261

Bisht, S., & Bist, S. S. (2011). Curcumin: A potential therapeutic agent for chronic inflammatory diseases. *Journal of Advanced Pharmaceutical Technology & Research*, 2(1), 11-18. https://doi.org/10.4103/2231-4040.79796

Chaganti, R. K., & Felson, D. T. (2013). Nutritional factors and osteoarthritis: A review. *Current Opinion in Rheumatology*, 25(1), 80-85. https://doi.org/10.1097/BOR.0b013e32835a941d

Felson, D. T. (2010). Osteoarthritis as a disease of mechanics. *Osteoarthritis and Cartilage*, 18(3), 305-310. https://doi.org/10.1016/j.joca.2009.12.008

Henrotin, Y., Lambert, C., Couchourel, D., Ripoll, C., & Chiotelli, E. (2011). Nutraceuticals: Do they represent a new era in the management of osteoarthritis? A narrative review from the lessons taken with five products. *Osteoarthritis and Cartilage*, 19(1), 1-21. https://doi.org/10.1016/j.joca.2010.10.017

Leech, R. M., McNaughton, S. A., & Worsley, A. (2015). The role of energy balance in the prevention and management of osteoarthritis. *Obesity Reviews*, 16(7), 557-571. https://doi.org/10.1111/obr.12285

Perricone, C., Bartoloni, E., Bursi, R., et al. (2015). Mediterranean diet and prevention of chronic diseases. *Clinical Reviews in Allergy & Immunology*, 50(1), 1-22. https://doi.org/10.1007/s12016-015-8497-8

Shapiro, B. H., & Principe, M. F. (2015). The role of dietary supplements in osteoarthritis: Current evidence and recommendations. *Journal of Clinical Rheumatology*, 21(8), 451-457. https://doi.org/10.1097/RHU.0000000000000304

Zhuo, Q., Yang, W., Chen, J., & Wang, Y. (2012). Metabolic syndrome meets osteoarthritis. *Nature Reviews Rheumatology*, 8(12), 729-737. https://doi.org/10.1038/nrrheum.2012.135

9. Psychological and behavioural therapies

9.1 Significance of psychosocial factors in osteoarthritis

9.1.1 Influence of stress, depression and anxiety on the course of the disease

Psychosocial factors play a central role in chronic diseases such as osteoarthritis. The reciprocal relationship between psychological stress and the experience of pain is well documented.

Chronic stress leads to the activation of the hypothalamic-pituitary-adrenal axis (HPA axis) and the release of stress hormones such as cortisol. Prolonged activation of these systems can intensify the perception of pain, reduce pain tolerance and promote inflammatory activity in the body.

Depressive moods and anxiety disorders are particularly common in osteoarthritis patients. The persistent pain, loss of mobility and the associated reduction in quality of life favour the occurrence of psychological comorbidities.

Conversely, depression and anxiety worsen the subjective perception of pain and promote the development of passive illness behaviour, which increases physical inactivity and social isolation.

9.1.2 Cognitive distortions and their effects on pain perception

Cognitive distortions such as catastrophising and selective perception reinforce the negative evaluation of pain and promote dysfunctional behavioural patterns.

Catastrophising is characterised by the constant expectation that the pain will increase or can no longer be controlled. This leads to an increased emotional reaction to pain stimuli and to greater activation of pain-processing areas in the brain.

The so-called "fear-avoidance behaviour" is also frequently observed in osteoarthritis patients. Fear of pain leads to avoidance of exercise, even though moderate physical activity has been proven to help relieve pain.

These negative thought and behaviour patterns contribute significantly to the chronification of pain and make it difficult to successfully implement treatment plans.

9.2 Psychotherapeutic approaches in osteoarthritis therapy

9.2.1 Cognitive behavioural therapy (CBT)

Cognitive behavioural therapy is one of the best-studied psychotherapeutic methods in pain therapy.

The aims of CBT are

- Recognising and changing dysfunctional thought patterns that negatively influence the perception of pain.
- Development of adaptive coping strategies to improve dealing with pain.
- Promoting active problem-solving strategies and positive coping with illness.

Various therapeutic methods are used, including

- Cognitive restructuring to identify and change catastrophising thoughts.
- Relaxation techniques to reduce stress, such as progressive muscle relaxation or breathing techniques.
- Behavioural experiments to experience the positive effect of movement and activity despite pain.

Numerous studies have shown that CBT reduces the perception of pain, reduces emotional stress and significantly improves quality of life.

9.2.2 Acceptance and Commitment Therapy (ACT)

Acceptance and commitment therapy is a modern psychotherapeutic approach that supports patients in developing a different way of dealing with chronic pain.

In contrast to cognitive behavioural therapy, the focus is not on directly changing thoughts, but on accepting painful experiences without allowing them to dominate actions.

ACT pursues the following goals:

- Promoting mental flexibility in order to lead a fulfilling life despite pain.
- Develop a mindful attitude towards painful thoughts and feelings.
- Emphasising values and aligning one's own actions with these values, regardless of the pain symptoms.

ACT has proven to be particularly effective for patients with chronic pain syndromes that are difficult to treat and is increasingly being integrated into multimodal pain therapy concepts.

9.3 Relaxation techniques and mindfulness training

9.3.1 Progressive muscle relaxation according to Jacobson

Progressive muscle relaxation (PMR) is one of the most widely used relaxation techniques and was developed by Edmund Jacobson back in the 1930s.

It is based on the principle that a state of deep physical and mental relaxation can be achieved by consciously tensing and then relaxing various muscle groups.

Systematic execution leads to a reduction in sympathetic activity, a decrease in muscle tension and improved blood flow to the muscles and joints.

The advantage of PMR for osteoarthritis patients is that they can actively regulate the tension that often arises from chronic pain. Studies show that regular use not only reduces the perception of pain, but also improves sleep quality and general well-being.

9.3.2 Mindfulness and meditation: MBSR programmes

The Mindfulness-Based Stress Reduction programme (MBSR) was developed by Jon Kabat-Zinn and combines meditative mindfulness exercises with gentle movement and body awareness.

The aim is to develop a conscious and non-judgemental approach to physical sensations, thoughts and emotions.

Patients learn to observe pain and discomfort without reflexively judging or avoiding them. This altered perception leads to less emotional reactivity to pain stimuli and can significantly reduce the intensity of chronic pain.

Studies show that MBSR programmes significantly improve quality of life, pain tolerance and psychological well-being in chronic pain conditions such as osteoarthritis.

9.3.3 Biofeedback and its application for chronic pain

Biofeedback is a scientifically recognised procedure in which physiological processes such as heart rate, muscle tension, breathing rate or skin conductivity are visualised using technical devices.

By receiving direct feedback, patients can learn to influence their physical reactions in a targeted manner.

In osteoarthritis therapy, biofeedback is used in particular to:

- Reduce muscular tension in the area of the joint-stabilising muscles.
- To promote conscious control over breathing and relaxation reactions.
- To reduce chronic pain reactions through controlled regulation of the autonomic nervous system.

In the long term, biofeedback can strengthen self-efficacy and help patients to take an active role in coping with pain.

9.4 Educational programmes and self-management

9.4.1 Patient education for pain management

A central element of modern osteoarthritis therapy is the comprehensive education of patients about the disease mechanisms, the course of the disease and the realistic treatment goals.

Convey educational programmes:

- Basic knowledge of the pathophysiology of osteoarthritis.
- Strategies for independent pain control and functional improvement.

- Dealing with psychosocial stress and promoting positive coping with illness.

Through targeted training, patients can be encouraged to take responsibility for their health, increase their own activity and recognise and change harmful behaviour patterns.

9.4.2 Development of coping strategies and pain competence

Developing a high level of pain competence is crucial to prevent pain from becoming chronic.

Central coping strategies include

- Cognitive strategies such as the positive reinterpretation of stressful situations.
- Active problem-solving strategies for the targeted management of everyday limitations.
- Social support and the conscious development of positive social contacts.
- Emotional regulation through relaxation and mindfulness techniques.

A well-developed self-management programme helps to overcome the helplessness that often accompanies chronic illnesses and to significantly improve quality of life even if the illness persists.

9.5 Bibliography (Chapter 9)

Andersson, G., & Turk, D. C. (2014). The psychology of chronic pain: The relevance and implications for treatment. *Current Opinion in Psychiatry*, 27(5), 370-375. https://doi.org/10.1097/YCO.0000000000000092

Baer, R. A. (2003). Mindfulness training as a clinical intervention: A conceptual and empirical review. *Clinical Psychology: Science and Practice*, 10(2), 125-143. https://doi.org/10.1093/clipsy/bpg015

Cohen, M. J., Quintner, J. L., & Buchanan, D. (2013). Is chronic pain a disease? *Pain Medicine*, 14(9), 1284-1289. https://doi.org/10.1111/pme.12114

Eccleston, C., Morley, S., & Williams, A. (2013). Psychological approaches to chronic pain management: Evidence and challenges. *British Journal of Anaesthesia*, 111(1), 59-63. https://doi.org/10.1093/bja/aet109

Kabat-Zinn, J. (1990). *Full Catastrophe Living: Using the Wisdom of Your Body and Mind to Face Stress, Pain, and Illness*. New York: Delacorte.

Keefe, F. J., Main, C. J., & George, S. Z. (2018). Advancing psychologically informed practice for patients with persistent musculoskeletal pain: Promise, pitfalls, and solutions. *Physical Therapy*, 98(5), 398-407. https://doi.org/10.1093/ptj/pzy034

McCracken, L. M., & Vowles, K. E. (2014). Acceptance and commitment therapy and mindfulness for chronic pain: Model, process, and progress. *American Psychologist*, 69(2), 178-187. https://doi.org/10.1037/a0035623

Morley, S., & Williams, A. (2015). New developments in the psychological management of chronic pain. *Canadian Journal of Psychiatry*, 60(4), 168-175.
https://doi.org/10.1177/070674371506000403

Turk, D. C., & Okifuji, A. (2010). Psychological factors in chronic pain: Evolution and revolution. *Journal of Consulting and Clinical Psychology*, 70(3), 678-690.
https://doi.org/10.1037/0022-006X.70.3.678

Veehof, M. M., Oskam, M. J., Schreurs, K. M., & Bohlmeijer, E. T. (2011). Acceptance-based interventions for the treatment of chronic pain: A systematic review and meta-analysis. *Pain*, 152(3), 533-542.
https://doi.org/10.1016/j.pain.2010.11.002

10. Interdisciplinary and multimodal treatment concepts

10.1 The need for an integrative therapeutic approach

10.1.1 Limits of monotherapeutic interventions

For a long time, the treatment of osteoarthritis was characterised by a monotherapeutic approach, with the focus on either medication, physiotherapy or surgery.

However, these one-sided treatment strategies often fall short, as osteoarthritis is a complex disease that encompasses structural, functional and psychosocial aspects.

Focusing solely on symptomatic pain therapy without considering the underlying biomechanical, metabolic and psychological factors may help to alleviate symptoms in the short term, but rarely leads to a lasting improvement in quality of life or stabilisation of the course of the disease.

Patients with advanced stages of the disease, multiple comorbidities and chronic pain in particular do not benefit sufficiently from isolated treatment approaches.

10.1.2 Advantages of combined forms of therapy

An integrative, multimodal treatment concept combines various therapeutic measures that address the physical as well as the psychological and social factors influencing the disease.

The main advantages of such concepts include

- Improvement of pain control through the use of synergistic therapy elements.

- Increasing functional ability and mobility through coordinated rehabilitation measures.

- Reduction of medication consumption and thus of side effects through complementary non-drug treatments.

- Sustainable improvement in mental health and quality of life through targeted psychotherapeutic and educational interventions.

Multimodal programmes are also increasingly being implemented in specialist pain clinics and rehabilitation centres in order to provide holistic and individualised care for complex cases of osteoarthritis.

10.2 Models of multimodal pain therapy

10.2.1 Design and structure of multimodal programmes

Multimodal pain therapy programmes are generally interdisciplinary in nature and involve close cooperation between various specialist areas, including

- Orthopaedics and rheumatology
- Pain medicine

- Physiotherapy and sports medicine
- Psychotherapy and behavioural therapy
- Nutritional counselling

The duration of treatment varies depending on the severity of the disease, but programmes are usually carried out over several weeks with daily therapy sessions.

A typical day includes:

- Medical rounds and pain therapy
- Physiotherapy and exercise therapy to improve joint function
- Psychological group sessions for pain management and stress management
- Relaxation techniques and mindfulness training
- Nutritional training and personalised advice

10.2.2 Evidence and success of interdisciplinary approaches

Numerous studies have proven the effectiveness of multimodal concepts for chronic pain disorders, including osteoarthritis.

Meta-analyses show significant improvements in the following areas:

- Reduction of pain intensity

- Increase in physical functionality
- Improving mental health and reducing depression and anxiety disorders
- Long-term reduction in the use of drug therapies

Multimodal approaches are now considered the gold standard in the treatment of complex chronic pain disorders and are expressly recommended by international guidelines such as those of the OARSI (Osteoarthritis Research Society International).

10.3 Integration of innovative therapies into established treatment concepts

10.3.1 Use of biological and cellular therapies as part of multimodal programmes

The increasing availability of biological and cellular therapies, such as stem cell therapy, chondrocyte transplantation or the use of exosomes, represents a promising expansion of multimodal osteoarthritis treatment programmes.

These innovative procedures offer the possibility of regenerating structural damage to the joint cartilage in a targeted manner and halting degenerative processes.

However, in order to maximise the benefits of these approaches, it is crucial that they are not used in isolation, but as an integral part of a comprehensive therapy concept.

The optimum procedure is as follows:

- Targeted diagnostics to identify suitable candidates for biological therapies.

- Combination of cell-based therapies with a structured rehabilitation programme to optimally control the mechanical loads on the joint.

- Supplementary physical therapy to promote tissue regeneration and improve joint stability.

The post-therapeutic phase after cellular interventions should be accompanied by regular check-ups in order to objectively assess the success of the measures and to be able to react to possible complications in good time.

10.3.2 Combination of classic and innovative therapeutic approaches

The successful treatment of osteoarthritis often requires a combination of proven conventional methods and innovative new approaches.

For example, a patient may benefit from initial pain control through pharmacological measures and physical applications in order to subsequently undergo regenerative therapy such as stem cell injection or matrix-associated chondrocyte implantation.

In the further course of treatment, physiotherapeutic measures are then used to stabilise the joint, psychotherapeutic interventions to improve pain management and educational programmes to support active self-management.

Such dynamic and customised therapy planning can achieve both short-term relief of symptoms and long-term improvement in joint function and quality of life.

10.4 Challenges and prospects for integrative care

10.4.1 Organisational and economic hurdles

The implementation of interdisciplinary and multimodal treatment concepts is associated with considerable organisational and economic challenges.

The most common barriers include

- High personnel and logistical effort to coordinate the various specialist disciplines.

- Lack of networking between outpatient and inpatient care.

- Insufficient reimbursement of multimodal therapy programmes by health insurance providers, especially for innovative therapies that are not yet widely approved.

- Limited capacity of specialised facilities that can offer comprehensive multimodal care.

In the long term, health policy initiatives are needed to anchor the importance of these holistic approaches more firmly in the healthcare system and to ensure their sustainable funding.

10.4.2 Future prospects for interdisciplinary osteoarthritis treatment

The future of osteoarthritis therapy undoubtedly lies in the consistent implementation of integrative care concepts.

The increasing establishment of specialist centres for musculoskeletal diseases, the digitalisation of care processes and the use of modern telemedicine services will make it easier to coordinate complex treatment programmes efficiently in the future.

In addition, the growing evidence on the positive effects of multimodal approaches will help to ensure that these forms of treatment are more closely integrated into guidelines and reimbursement systems.

The close integration of research, clinical practice and patient participation will be a key success factor in developing and permanently establishing individualised, effective and economically viable therapy concepts.

10.5   Bibliography (Chapter 10)

Bannuru, R. R., Osani, M. C., Vaysbrot, E. E., et al. (2019). OARSI guidelines for the non-surgical management of knee, hip, and polyarticular osteoarthritis. *Osteoarthritis and Cartilage*,

27(11), 1578-1589. https://doi.org/10.1016/j.joca.2019.06.011

Dagenais, S., Caro, J., & Haldeman, S. (2008). A systematic review of low back pain cost of illness studies in the United States and internationally. *Spine Journal*, 8(1), 8-20. https://doi.org/10.1016/j.spinee.2007.10.005

Gatchel, R. J., Peng, Y. B., Peters, M. L., Fuchs, P. N., & Turk, D. C. (2007). The biopsychosocial approach to chronic pain: Scientific advances and future directions. *Psychological Bulletin*, 133(4), 581-624. https://doi.org/10.1037/0033-2909.133.4.581

Hoffman, B. M., Papas, R. K., Chatkoff, D. K., & Kerns, R. D. (2007). Meta-analysis of psychological interventions for chronic low back pain. *Health Psychology*, 26(1), 1-9. https://doi.org/10.1037/0278-6133.26.1.1

Hooten, W. M. (2016). Chronic pain and mental health disorders: Shared neural mechanisms, epidemiology, and treatment. *Mayo Clinic Proceedings*, 91(7), 955-970. https://doi.org/10.1016/j.mayocp.2016.02.018

Karjalainen, K., Malmivaara, A., van Tulder, M., et al. (2001). Multidisciplinary biopsychosocial rehabilitation for subacute low back pain in working-age adults. *Cochrane Database of Systematic Reviews*, (2), CD002193. https://doi.org/10.1002/14651858.CD002193

Klinger, R., Blasini, M., Schmitz, J., & Colloca, L. (2018). Nocebo effects in clinical studies: Hints for pain therapy.

Pain Reports, 3(3), e654. https://doi.org/10.1097/PR9.0000000000000654

Turk, D. C., Wilson, H. D., & Cahana, A. (2011). Treatment of chronic non-cancer pain. *The Lancet*, 377(9784), 2226-2235. https://doi.org/10.1016/S0140-6736(11)60402-9

Von Korff, M., & Moore, J. C. (2001). Stepped care for back pain: Activating self-care. *Spine*, 26(24), 2671-2679. https://doi.org/10.1097/00007632-200112150-00007

Wetherell, J. L., Afari, N., Rutledge, T., et al. (2011). Acceptance and commitment therapy for generalised anxiety disorder: A pilot study. *Behaviour Therapy*, 42(1), 56-68. https://doi.org/10.1016/j.beth.2010.03.002

11. Personalised medicine and genetic therapy approaches

11.1 Basics of personalised osteoarthritis therapy

11.1.1 Significance of genetic predispositions for the risk of disease

The development and progression of osteoarthritis is a complex multifactorial process resulting from the interaction of genetic predispositions, molecular biological mechanisms and a wide range of environmental influences. This close interweaving of biological and external factors means that both the risk of developing the disease and its clinical course can vary considerably from individual to individual. While environmental factors such as mechanical stress, obesity or injuries play an important role, the significance of genetic predispositions is increasingly becoming the focus of scientific research, as they exert a fundamental influence on individual susceptibility to osteoarthritic changes.

In recent years, extensive genome-wide association studies (GWAS) have identified a number of genetic variants that are significantly associated with an increased risk of developing osteoarthritis. These genetic factors primarily influence the structure, function and regenerative capacity of articular cartilage, subchondral bone and connective tissue. Gene variations that directly intervene in the regulation of collagen, matrix metalloproteinases and growth and differentiation processes are particularly noteworthy.

Important genetic risk factors include

- Polymorphisms in the **COL2A1 gene**, which codes for collagen type II. Type II collagen is the main component of articular cartilage and is crucial for its mechanical stability and resilience. Mutations or polymorphisms in this gene can lead to a structural weakening of the cartilage, which significantly increases susceptibility to degenerative changes.

- Gene variants in the **MMP-13 gene**, which regulates the expression of matrix metalloproteinases, in particular MMP-13. MMP-13 is an enzyme that is significantly involved in the degradation of the extracellular matrix and in particular promotes the degradation of collagen type II in articular cartilage. Overactivation of this enzyme leads to accelerated cartilage degeneration, which is a central pathophysiological feature of osteoarthritis.

- variants in the **GDF5 gene** (Growth Differentiation Factor 5), which plays a key role in chondrogenesis and the development of articular cartilage. GDF5 is a growth factor that promotes the differentiation of mesenchymal stem cells into chondrocytes and thus significantly supports the formation and regeneration of cartilage tissue. Genetic variants that impair the expression or function of GDF5 can significantly reduce the ability to regenerate cartilage.

The identification of such genetic risk factors is of central importance for early risk stratification. It makes it possible to recognise potentially at-risk individuals at a preclinical stage and provide targeted information. In addition, knowledge of genetic predispositions opens up new avenues for preventive measures and individualised therapeutic strategies that are tailored to the specific molecular causes of the disease. In the long term, the integration of genetic diagnostics into clinical practice can help to positively influence the course of the disease and significantly improve the quality of life of affected patients.

11.1.2 Biomarkers for therapy customisation and prognosis assessment

The use of biomarkers in the diagnosis and treatment planning of osteoarthritis has become considerably more important in recent years. Biomarkers are measurable biological parameters that provide objective information about physiological or pathophysiological processes and serve as the basis for a more precise classification of the disease, the selection of individualised treatment options and the assessment of prognosis. The integration of biomarkers into clinical decision-making represents a decisive step towards personalised medicine, which makes it possible to optimally adapt treatment strategies to the individual needs and risk profiles of patients.

The most important biomarkers in the context of osteoarthritis include

- **Inflammatory markers**, including in particular C-reactive protein (CRP) and interleukin-6 (IL-6). CRP is an acute-phase protein whose concentration in the blood plasma rises rapidly during systemic inflammatory reactions. An elevated CRP level may indicate inflammatory processes associated with osteoarthritis, even if the disease is primarily degenerative in nature. IL-6 is a pro-inflammatory cytokine that plays a central role in the activation and maintenance of inflammatory processes. Elevated IL-6 levels are often associated with active disease progression and a poorer prognosis.

- **Cartilage degradation products**, in particular collagen type II degradation products (CTX-II), which are detectable in urine. These biomarkers reflect the current status of cartilage degradation and provide information about the catabolic activities in the joint. An elevated CTX-II level is often regarded as an indicator of progressive joint destruction and can be used to assess the stage of the disease and to monitor the success of treatment.

- **Genetic markers** that are primarily used in the form of SNP analyses (single nucleotide polymorphisms). These analyses enable the identification of genetic risk profiles that are associated with an increased susceptibility to the development and progression of osteoarthritis. By recording such genetic markers, the individual disease prognosis can be assessed more precisely and a targeted selection of therapeutic interventions can be made.

The use of biomarkers not only allows a more differentiated diagnosis to be made, but also opens up the possibility of monitoring the course of the disease at a molecular biological level and reacting to therapeutic changes or deteriorations in the clinical condition at an early stage. Biomarkers also make a significant contribution to the development of new drugs, as they can be used as surrogate endpoints in clinical trials to assess the efficacy and safety of innovative therapeutic approaches.

In the long term, the targeted use of biomarkers is expected to become an integral part of personalised osteoarthritis treatment. This will not only make treatment more efficient, but will also significantly improve patients' quality of life through early and needs-based intervention.

11.2 Genetic diagnostics and individual risk profiles

11.2.1 Methods of genome analysis in osteoarthritis research

Modern genome research has made significant progress in recent years through the use of high-resolution molecular genetic analysis methods, which have also significantly advanced research into complex degenerative diseases such as osteoarthritis. At the centre of this development is next-generation sequencing (NGS) technology, which enables in-depth and comprehensive analysis of large sections of the genome at high speed and cost-effectively. This technology is revolutionising genetic diagnostics, as it allows a considerable increase in the amount of data compared to conventional sequencing methods while simultaneously reducing costs and dramatically shortening analysis times.

NGS technology makes it possible to analyse the entire genome as well as targeted sections such as the exome or specific regulatory regions of the DNA in detail. This enables the systematic identification of genetic variants that may be associated with an increased susceptibility to osteoarthritis or a specific course of the disease. These findings contribute significantly to a better understanding of the pathophysiological basis of osteoarthritis and to the development of new therapeutic approaches based on the individual genetic risk factors of patients.

Particularly relevant methods of analysis in osteoarthritis research are:

- **Whole exome sequencing (WES)**: This method focuses on analysing the coding sections of the genome, i.e. the exons that are responsible for the synthesis of proteins. As many disease-relevant genetic variations directly influence protein structure and function, WES enables a targeted investigation of those gene regions that could be directly involved in the pathogenesis of osteoarthritis. By identifying pathogenic variants in genes that control, for example, cartilage homeostasis, bone metabolism or the regulation of inflammatory processes, a precise risk profile can be created.

- **SNP arrays (single nucleotide polymorphism arrays)**: This technology is used to identify known genetic risk variants that have already been associated with an increased risk of osteoarthritis in the scientific literature. By analysing hundreds of thousands to millions of individual nucleotide variations in the genome, risk genes can be identified quickly and efficiently. This method is particularly suitable for population-based studies and the creation of genetic risk maps, which enable a more precise assessment of individual disease risk.

- **Epigenetic analyses:** In addition to the direct analysis of the DNA sequence, epigenetic analyses are becoming increasingly important. The focus here is particularly on DNA methylation patterns that regulate gene expression without changing the underlying nucleotide sequence. Changes in the methylation of genes that are involved in the regulation of inflammatory processes or cartilage metabolism, for example, can contribute significantly to the development and progression of osteoarthritis. Epigenetic markers therefore offer an additional, important dimension for the creation of individual risk profiles and the development of new therapeutic approaches that specifically influence epigenetic modifications.

The application of these state-of-the-art genetic and epigenetic analysis methods enables a comprehensive characterisation of the individual genetic disposition of osteoarthritis patients. These findings form the scientific basis for the development of personalised prevention and treatment strategies that are specifically tailored to the molecular biological characteristics of each patient.

11.2.2 Development of personalised prevention and treatment strategies

Knowledge of individual genetic risk factors opens up completely new perspectives in the prevention and treatment of osteoarthritis. By identifying genetic predispositions at an early stage, preventive measures can be introduced with the aim of delaying the onset of the disease or, ideally, preventing it altogether. This represents a paradigmatic shift in medical care from reactive treatment to a proactive, preventative approach.

Long before clinically manifest symptoms of osteoarthritis appear, an individual risk assessment can be carried out by analysing genetic risk profiles. Based on this risk assessment, targeted measures can be recommended that affect both lifestyle and medical care.

These preventive and therapeutic measures include, among others:

- **Early recommendations for reducing mechanical stress**: In the case of genetically determined weaknesses of the cartilage tissue, for example due to proven polymorphisms in the COL2A1 gene, a targeted reduction of excessive joint loads is essential. Individually adapted training and exercise programmes that relieve the joints and at the same time promote muscular stabilisation help to slow down degenerative processes and maintain joint function in the long term.

- **Specific nutritional and micronutrient recommendations**: The targeted intake of nutrients that support cartilage homeostasis plays a central role in the prevention and treatment of osteoarthritis. These include in particular substances such as omega-3 fatty acids, antioxidants, vitamin D, vitamin K2 and certain amino acids, which have been shown to have anti-inflammatory and cartilage-protective properties. In the case of known genetic risk profiles, these recommendations can be customised to specifically support cartilage metabolism.

- Selection of therapy options that specifically influence molecular disease mechanisms: Depending on the genetic risk factors identified, therapy can be targeted at specific pathophysiological mechanisms. For example, the use of MMP-13 inhibitors can be considered to slow down cartilage degradation if the MMP-13 gene is found to be overactive. The use of biological therapies that specifically inhibit pro-inflammatory cytokines can also be useful, depending on the individual genetic profile.

In clinical practice, this personalised approach is increasingly being supplemented by the combination of genetic diagnostics with conventional imaging such as magnetic resonance imaging (MRI) and laboratory chemical parameters. This integrative diagnostics enables a comprehensive assessment of the current stage of the disease and a differentiated treatment plan tailored to the molecular and clinical findings.

In the long term, personalised medicine will permanently change osteoarthritis treatment by enabling greater therapeutic efficacy with fewer side effects. Targeted prevention and individualised therapy planning can not only slow down the progression of the disease, but also significantly improve patients' quality of life and substantially reduce the social costs associated with the treatment and care of osteoarthritis patients.

11.3 Gene therapy and molecular interventions

11.3.1 Possibilities of targeted gene modification (CRISPR/Cas9 and other methods)

Gene therapy opens up completely new therapeutic perspectives in the field of osteoarthritis treatment, as it directly addresses the molecular causes of the disease. Instead of merely alleviating the symptoms or slowing down the progression of the disease, gene therapy aims to correct pathological processes at a genetic level or even eliminate them completely. The most significant technological advance in this area to date is the development of **CRISPR/Cas9 technology**, which enables precise and comparatively simple modification of genetic material.

CRISPR/Cas9 is based on a natural defence mechanism of bacteria against viruses and has been adapted for targeted genome editing in human and animal cells. This method allows disease-causing genes to be specifically switched off (**knockout**) or protective genes to be specifically activated or new functional genes to be inserted (**knock-in**). The high precision and efficiency of this method makes it particularly attractive for the research and potential treatment of genetic degenerative diseases such as osteoarthritis.

In current osteoarthritis research, CRISPR technology is primarily used for the following targeted therapeutic approaches:

- Inhibition of the expression of cartilage-degrading enzymes, in particular **matrix metalloproteinase-13 (MMP-13)**. This enzyme plays a central role in the catabolic degradation process of articular cartilage by degrading the main component of the cartilage matrix, collagen type II. By specifically inactivating the MMP-13 gene, cartilage degeneration can be significantly slowed down or even prevented.

- **Blocking the production of pro-inflammatory cytokines**, in particular **interleukin-1β (IL-1β)**, which plays a key role in maintaining chronic inflammatory processes in the joint. Genetic deactivation of the IL-1β gene reduces the inflammatory component of osteoarthritis, which can have a favourable effect on the course of the disease.

- **Enhancement of the chondroprotective effect of genes such as SOX9**, one of the most important transcription factors for the differentiation and function of chondrocytes. SOX9 promotes the synthesis of cartilage matrix components and supports the regeneration of cartilage tissue. Targeted overexpression of SOX9 could significantly improve the self-healing capacity of cartilage and halt degenerative processes.

In addition to CRISPR/Cas9, other methods of targeted gene modification are also used, such as **zinc finger nucleases (ZFNs)** and **transcription activator-like effector nucleases (TALENs)**. These technologies are based on the specific recognition of DNA sequences by artificially constructed proteins that bind to defined sites in the genome and trigger targeted DNA strand breaks there. However, these methods are less precise than CRISPR/Cas9, are technically more complex and have a higher risk of so-called off-target effects, in which genetic changes are unintentionally triggered at unintended sites in the genome. For these reasons, their use in clinical practice has so far remained limited.

In future, the further development of these technologies will primarily aim to further increase precision, minimise off-target risks and ensure the long-term safety of genetic modifications. In particular, the combination of genome editing with modern carrier systems could significantly advance the clinical application of these innovative therapeutic approaches.

11.3.2 Use of viral vectors and non-viral carrier systems

A central problem in the application of genetic therapies is the safe and efficient transfer of the therapeutic genes into the target cells. As the isolated administration of DNA or RNA does not usually lead to sufficient uptake into the cells, specialised **carrier systems (vectors)** are required to support the transfer of genetic information. A distinction is made between **viral** and **non-viral** vector systems, each of which has specific advantages and disadvantages.

- Viral vectors:
Viral systems utilise the natural ability of viruses to introduce genetic material into host cells. The most frequently used vectors in osteoarthritis research include **adeno-associated viruses (AAV)** and **lentiviruses**.

AAVs are characterised by high transfection efficiency, comparatively low immunogenicity and preferential uptake into certain tissues, including joint tissue. A major advantage of AAVs is the low integration of their genetic material into the host genome, which reduces the risk of unintentional genome modification.

Lentiviruses, on the other hand, are able to permanently integrate their genetic material into the host genome. This enables long-lasting expression of therapeutic genes, but also harbours the risk of **insertional mutagenesis**, in which random integration into the genome can disrupt the function of important genes and possibly lead to uncontrolled cell proliferation or even tumour development.

Despite these risks, viral vectors are currently recognised as the most effective systems for gene delivery into joint tissue due to their high efficiency and targeting. Intensive research is focused on controlling the immunological responses to viral vectors and further improving the safety of these approaches.

- Non-viral vectors:
Non-viral systems include a wide range of synthetic carriers, such as **liposomes, polymer nanoparticles** and **plasmid DNA systems**. These carrier systems have the major advantage of low immunogenicity and better control of pharmacokinetic properties. They also carry no risk of uncontrolled integration into the host genome, which means that serious side effects such as tumour development can be avoided.

However, non-viral carrier systems have so far been clearly limited in their efficiency of gene transfer. The uptake of the genetic material into the target cells is often inadequate and the expression of the therapeutic genes achieved is usually transient and quantitatively limited. In addition, these systems have so far lacked a pronounced tissue specificity, which can lead to an unspecific distribution of the therapeutic genes in the body.

Future development will therefore focus on optimising these carrier systems in order to enable the targeted, efficient and, above all, safe transfer of therapeutic genes. Among other things, multifunctional nanoparticles are being developed that are equipped with surface molecules that enable targeted binding to specific cell types in the joint tissue. In addition, innovative materials are being researched that ensure the controlled release of genetic information and can achieve a long-term therapeutic effect.

The combination of high-precision genome editing technologies such as CRISPR/Cas9 with advanced carrier systems represents a promising approach to making the personalised gene therapy of the future clinically usable for the treatment of osteoarthritis. Patient safety is the top priority here, which is why future clinical trials will be particularly focussed on a careful risk-benefit assessment and long-term monitoring of possible side effects.

11.4 Ethical implications of genetic therapy approaches

11.4.1 Weighing up medical progress and ethical concerns

The development and application of genetic therapies in the field of osteoarthritis raises far-reaching ethical questions.

While somatic gene therapies aimed at treating individual patients are ethically accepted in many countries, the manipulation of the human genome at germline level - i.e. interventions that can be passed on to subsequent generations - remains highly controversial from an ethical point of view.

Although somatic gene therapy is primarily relevant in the context of osteoarthritis, it is important to weigh up the risks carefully:

- How safe are the genome editing methods used in the long term?
- Can undesirable genetic changes ("off-target effects") be excluded?
- Is it justifiable to carry out irreversible interventions whose long-term consequences have not yet been sufficiently researched?

These questions must be discussed in detail and answered in accordance with ethical guidelines before genetic therapies can be widely used in clinical practice.

11.4.2 Regulatory framework and social acceptance

The use of genetic diagnostics and therapy is subject to strict legal regulations in most Western countries.

- In the European Union, Regulation (EC) No. 1394/2007 regulates the use of advanced therapy medicinal products (ATMPs), which also include gene and cell therapies.

- In Germany, gene therapy is also subject to the Genetic Engineering Act and the Medicinal Products Act, which stipulate extensive authorisation procedures and proof of safety.

- In the USA, the Food and Drug Administration (FDA) coordinates the authorisation of genetic therapies, which are also subject to high safety and efficacy standards.

The social acceptance of genetic methods depends to a large extent on the transparency of research, the open communication of opportunities and risks and compliance with ethical principles.

A broad social discourse is needed to ensure a balance between the legitimate interest in medical progress and the protection of individual rights and the integrity of future generations.

11.5 Bibliography (Chapter 11)

Attur, M., Krasnokutsky, S., & Abramson, S. B. (2010). Targeting the synovial tissue for treating osteoarthritis (OA): Where is the evidence? *Best Practice & Research Clinical Rheumatology*, 24(1), 71-79.
https://doi.org/10.1016/j.berh.2009.08.006

Evans, C. H., Ghivizzani, S. C., & Robbins, P. D. (2011). Gene transfer to human joints: Progress toward a gene therapy of arthritis. *Proceedings of the National Academy of Sciences*,

108(48), 19072-19077.
https://doi.org/10.1073/pnas.1108293108

Hunter, D. J., & Bierma-Zeinstra, S. (2019). Osteoarthritis. *The Lancet*, 393(10182), 1745-1759.
https://doi.org/10.1016/S0140-6736(19)30417-9

Kim, Y. S., Smoak, M. M., Melchiorri, A. J., & Mikos, A. G. (2020). Gene delivery for osteoarthritis therapy. *Journal of Controlled Release*, 317, 285-300.
https://doi.org/10.1016/j.jconrel.2019.11.010

Li, Y., Wang, Y., Chubinskaya, S., et al. (2016). Genetic susceptibility to osteoarthritis: Functional polymorphisms in key candidate genes. *Arthritis Research & Therapy*, 18(1), 1-13.
https://doi.org/10.1186/s13075-016-1131-1

Mendelsohn, A. R., & Larrick, J. W. (2017). CRISPR-Cas9 genome editing for therapeutic applications: Progress and challenges. *Current Molecular Medicine*, 17(2), 98-114.
https://doi.org/10.2174/1566524017666170123105211

Reardon, S. (2016). First CRISPR clinical trial gets green light from US panel. *Nature*, 531(7593), 560-560.
https://doi.org/10.1038/nature.2016.20137

Zeggini, E., Panoutsopoulou, K., Southam, L., et al. (2012). Identification of new susceptibility loci for osteoarthritis (arcOGEN): A genome-wide association study. *The Lancet*, 380(9844), 815-823. https://doi.org/10.1016/S0140-6736(12)60681-3

Zhou, Y., Li, Y., Wang, K., et al. (2019). The roles of genetic and epigenetic factors in the pathogenesis of osteoarthritis.

Journal of Bone and Mineral Metabolism, 37(1), 1-11.
https://doi.org/10.1007/s00774-018-0948-3

12. The need for surgical interventions

12.1 The current status of surgical procedures in osteo-arthritis therapy

Surgical interventions, in particular endoprosthetic fittings such as the use of knee or hip joint endoprostheses, have been considered a proven standard therapy for advanced osteoarthritis for decades. These procedures are primarily indicated when conservative measures have been exhausted and the patient's quality of life is severely impaired by persistent pain and significant functional limitations.

The number of joint replacement operations performed worldwide has risen continuously in recent years. In Germany, for example, more than 450,000 endoprosthetic operations are performed on knee and hip joints every year.

These figures show that surgical procedures continue to play a central role in the treatment of osteoarthritis. However, the limitations of these interventions must also be taken into account:

- The durability of endoprostheses is limited, which leads to revision operations, especially in younger patients.

- Surgical procedures are associated with considerable risks, including infections, thrombosis, loosening of prostheses and complications during the healing process.

- Functional success depends largely on the patient's individual physical constitution, aftercare and active co-operation.

12.2 The state of research: Can new therapies replace surgical interventions?

The development of modern conservative and regenerative treatment methods has made considerable progress in recent years.

Biological and regenerative therapies

- The use of mesenchymal stem cells, exosomes and growth factors opens up new perspectives for regenerating damaged joint cartilage and halting the progression of osteoarthritis.

- Initial clinical studies show that the use of these innovative therapies can delay or even avoid the need for surgical intervention, particularly in patients in the early and middle stages of osteoarthritis.

- However, the long-term effects of these therapies have not yet been conclusively assessed, and regenerative measures also reach their limits in the case of advanced structural joint damage.

High-tech physiotherapy and robot-assisted rehabilitation procedures

- Advances in medical training therapy, supported by robotic exoskeletons and computerised movement analysis, make it possible to specifically improve joint function and compensate for muscular imbalances.

- These measures help to reduce the biomechanical stress on the affected joints and alleviate the symptoms in the long term.

Innovative drug therapy approaches

- The development of highly specific monoclonal antibodies, epigenetics-based drugs and gene modulation shows that inflammatory processes and catabolic metabolic pathways in joint tissue can be specifically influenced.

- However, most of these treatment approaches are still in clinical trials or preclinical testing.

12.3 Realistic perspectives: Will operations be superfluous in the future?

The idea that operations to treat osteoarthritis will become completely superfluous in the near future is not scientifically realistic from today's perspective.

Therapeutic progress is considerable, and with early diagnosis and consistent application of innovative therapeutic procedures, the need for surgical intervention can be significantly delayed.

Nevertheless, surgical procedures remain indispensable, especially in the following situations:

- In advanced osteoarthritic joint changes with complete loss of cartilage structure and severe deformities.

- In patients for whom conservative and regenerative treatment approaches do not achieve sufficient pain relief and functional improvement despite adequate implementation.

- In old age, when the body's ability to regenerate is naturally very limited and the focus is on rapid functional gains.

In the long term, however, the importance of surgical interventions could decline considerably if research into and clinical implementation of biological, molecular and technical therapeutic procedures continue to progress at the current rate.

12.4 Conclusion: Between hope and realistic assessment

In recent years, modern osteoarthritis therapy has developed from a purely symptomatic treatment to a holistic, multimodal approach that integrates biological, molecular, psychological and technological procedures.

While this progress gives justified hope for a reduction in surgical interventions, the complete substitution of surgical measures remains unrealistic at present and also in the medium term.

The key lies in early diagnosis, the consistent implementation of preventive measures and the optimal utilisation of available innovative therapies.

Operations will be required less frequently in future - but they are not expected to become completely superfluous in the coming decades.

13. International research perspectives and future developments

13.1 Current global research initiatives for osteoarthritis treatment

International research in the field of osteoarthritis treatment is characterised by close interdisciplinary collaboration between medicine, biotechnology, pharmacy and materials science. Numerous large research alliances and international initiatives are dedicated to the development of innovative diagnostic and therapeutic approaches.

Particularly noteworthy are:

- The Osteoarthritis Research Society International (OARSI), which is dedicated to promoting evidence-based research and clinical practice.

- The NIH initiative "Accelerating Medicines Partnership for Osteoarthritis (AMP OA)", which specifically promotes the development of disease-modifying therapies.

- The European research programme Horizon Europe, which promotes regenerative therapies and personalised treatment strategies in particular.

The focus of these initiatives is on the early diagnosis of osteoarthritis, the development of disease-modifying drugs, research into regenerative procedures and the integration of new technologies such as artificial intelligence for therapy planning.

13.2 Technological innovations and their relevance for osteoarthritis treatment

13.2.1. Artificial intelligence in diagnostics and therapy planning

Artificial intelligence (AI) is increasingly finding its way into medical diagnostics and individualised therapy planning.

Deep learning algorithms are used to analyse radiological image data, genetic information and clinical progression data in order to:

- recognise early stages of osteoarthritis more precisely before clinical symptoms become manifest.
- Predict the course of the disease on an individual basis.
- Develop optimised treatment plans based on patient-specific risk factors and treatment responses.

AI-supported systems also offer great potential in the development of new drugs and biological therapies by recognising complex molecular relationships more quickly and modelling suitable therapeutic approaches.

13.2.2 Progress in biomaterial research for cartilage replacement

Research into bioactive and biocompatible materials has made considerable progress in recent years.

Innovative biomaterials enable the development of:

- Hydrogel-based cartilage implants that release growth-promoting factors and support cartilage regeneration.
- 3D-printed cartilage structures that can be customised and implanted.
- Nanomaterials that serve as carrier systems for drugs or growth factors and are specifically introduced into the damaged joint areas.

These developments offer promising prospects for replacing natural cartilage in the long term or significantly promoting its regeneration.

13.3 International clinical trials and their results

13.3.1 Comparison of international study results on innovative therapies

A comparison of current international clinical studies makes it clear that the effectiveness of innovative therapeutic procedures depends heavily on individual patient requirements, the stage of the disease and the consistent application of therapy standards.

While intensive research into genetic and cell-based procedures is being conducted in the USA and China, European research is focussing more on multimodal treatment approaches and the integration of regenerative therapies into existing care concepts.

Previous studies show:

- Stem cell therapies achieve significant pain relief and functional improvement in early to mid-stage patients, but are less effective in advanced joint destruction.

- Exosome therapies show promising anti-inflammatory and regenerative effects, but are still largely at the experimental stage.

- PRP injections are widely used around the world and have proven their effectiveness for short-term symptom relief, but are of limited use for long-term disease modification.

13.3.2 Development of international guidelines and therapy recommendations

The international standardisation of treatment guidelines makes a decisive contribution to improving the quality of osteoarthritis therapy worldwide.

The OARSI guidelines and the recommendations of the American College of Rheumatology (ACR) and the European League Against Rheumatism (EULAR) are increasingly focussing on an evidence-based, interdisciplinary therapeutic approach.

Future guidelines are expected to be strengthened:

- Consider the importance of personalised and genetic therapy approaches.

- Integrate regenerative and biological procedures more closely into standardised treatment plans.

- Give greater weight to the effectiveness of non-pharmacological measures such as nutritional therapy, exercise and psychological support.

13.4 Conclusion: International perspectives for improved osteoarthritis therapy

The global research landscape clearly shows that osteoarthritis therapy is facing a fundamental change.

While surgical interventions continue to play an important role in advanced disease, holistic, patient-specific and disease-modifying therapeutic approaches are increasingly coming to the fore.

Progress in the field of regenerative medicine, the use of artificial intelligence to optimise therapy and the development of personalised treatment strategies at genetic and molecular level are particularly forward-looking.

The international networking of research, clinical practice and health policy will play a central role in establishing these innovative therapeutic approaches in the care of broad patient groups and sustainably improving the quality of life of osteoarthritis patients worldwide.

13.5 Bibliography (Chapter 13)

- Aletaha, D., Neogi, T., Silman, A. J., et al. (2010). 2010 Rheumatoid arthritis classification criteria: An American College of Rheumatology/European League Against Rheumatism collaborative initiative. *Annals of the Rheumatic Diseases*, 69(9), 1580-1588. https://doi.org/10.1136/ard.2010.138461

- Evans, C. H., & Ghivizzani, S. C. (2016). Gene therapy for osteoarthritis: What next? *Arthritis & Rheumatology*, 68(1), 1-3. https://doi.org/10.1002/art.39456

- Hunter, D. J., & Bierma-Zeinstra, S. (2019). Osteoarthritis. *The Lancet*, 393(10182), 1745-1759. https://doi.org/10.1016/S0140-6736(19)30417-9

- Kim, Y. S., Smoak, M. M., Melchiorri, A. J., & Mikos, A. G. (2020). Gene delivery for osteoarthritis therapy. *Journal of Controlled Release*, 317, 285-300. https://doi.org/10.1016/j.jconrel.2019.11.010

- OARSI (2020). Osteoarthritis: Current research and treatment recommendations. *Osteoarthritis Research Society International Guidelines*. Retrieved from https://oarsi.org

- Reardon, S. (2016). First CRISPR clinical trial gets green light from US panel. *Nature*, 531(7593), 560-560. https://doi.org/10.1038/nature.2016.20137

- Zeggini, E., Panoutsopoulou, K., Southam, L., et al. (2012). Identification of new susceptibility loci for osteoarthritis (arcOGEN): A genome-wide association study. *The Lancet*, 380(9844), 815-823. https://doi.org/10.1016/S0140-6736(12)60681-3

- Zhang, W., Moskowitz, R. W., Nuki, G., et al. (2010). OARSI recommendations for the management of hip and knee osteoarthritis: Part III. *Osteoarthritis and Cartilage*, 18(4), 476-499. https://doi.org/10.1016/j.joca.2010.01.013

14. Concluding remarks and conclusion

Osteoarthritis, one of the most common chronic degenerative joint diseases in the world, still poses major challenges for modern medicine today. Despite decades of intensive research and numerous therapeutic innovations, a complete cure for this disease remains elusive.

Nevertheless, it is undeniable that progress in recent years has brought considerable improvements in diagnostics, prevention, symptomatic treatment and especially in the development of regenerative and molecular therapy concepts.

The systematic further development of biological procedures such as stem cell therapy, the use of highly specific monoclonal antibodies, the application of innovative forms of physical therapy and the integration of genetic and epigenetic findings are opening up completely new horizons in the treatment of osteoarthritis.

The increasing interdisciplinary exchange between orthopaedics, pain therapy, molecular medicine, nutritional sciences and psychology is also contributing to a more comprehensive understanding of the complex pathophysiology of this disease.

Whereas in the past, the treatment of osteoarthritis was almost exclusively focussed on relieving pain and maintaining minimal joint function, today the focus is on holistically improving the quality of life, preventing the progression of the disease and, in an increasing number of cases, even partially regenerating damaged joint tissue.

The realisation that psychosocial factors, individual genetic dispositions, lifestyle and diet have a significant influence on the course of the disease has expanded the therapeutic approach from a purely symptomatic therapy to a comprehensive biopsychosocial treatment concept.

People are considered in their entirety - not just as carriers of a joint disease, but as complex beings with physical, psychological and social needs.

The coming years will show to what extent the innovative therapeutic approaches currently undergoing clinical and preclinical research have the potential to push joint replacement surgery further into the background or even make it superfluous.

One thing is already certain today: the earlier osteoarthritis is recognised and treated and the more consistently modern, evidence-based treatment methods are applied, the greater the chance of avoiding surgery in the long term and maintaining a stable quality of life.

The treatment of osteoarthritis is at a turning point. Whereas just a few decades ago only pain relief and joint replacement were considered treatment options, today there is an impressive range of therapeutic options available that have the potential to fundamentally influence the course of the disease.

However, this development is not a free pass for passive disease management. Rather, the successful application of modern therapies requires a high degree of personal responsibility, close interdisciplinary co-operation and the willingness to critically examine and sensibly integrate new scientific findings.

Surgery will continue to be necessary in many cases, especially with advanced disease. However, the proportion of patients for whom surgery can be avoided or significantly delayed thanks to innovative treatment strategies will continue to grow.

The major goal remains: To establish an effective therapy that has as few side effects as possible and is tailored to the individual needs of the patient, which improves the quality of life, slows down the progression of the disease and ultimately enables natural joint function to be maintained for as long as possible.

The future of osteoarthritis therapy is promising - but it also requires a responsible approach to the new possibilities and continuous scientific development. Only in this way will it be possible to realise the full potential of modern medicine in the service of those affected.

15 Table 1: Comparison of conventional and innovative osteoarthritis treatments

Criterion	Conventional therapy	Innovative therapy
Objective	Symptom relief	Disease modification
Forms of therapy	Painkillers, physiotherapy, operations	Stem cell therapy, exosomes, gene modulation
Onset of action	Short term	Medium to long term
Side effects	Frequent (e.g. gastrointestinal, cardiovascular)	Low, often experimental
Chances of recovery	No cure, symptomatic	Partial regeneration possible
Costs	Mainly refundable	High, often for private wear
Long-term success	Frequently limited	Potentially stabilising
Field of application	Advanced stages	Early to middle stage

16 Table 2: Most important micronutrients in osteoarthritis therapy

Micronutrient	Function in the organism	Effect on osteoarthritis	Recommended intake
Vitamin D	Bone metabolism, immunomodulation	Anti-inflammatory, bone-strengthening	800-2000 I.U./day
Vitamin C	Collagen synthesis, antioxidant	Protection of cartilage from oxidative stress	100-200 mg/day
Omega-3 fatty acids	Inflammation inhibition	Reduction of inflammatory mediators	1.5-3 g/day (EPA/DHA)
Zinc	Enzyme function, immunomodulation	Promotion of cartilage regeneration	10-15 mg/day
Selenium	Antioxidant cell protection	Reduction of oxidative stress	55-70 µg/day
Manganese	Cartilage formation, enzyme activity	Stabilisation of the cartilage matrix	2-5 mg/day

17 Table 3: Overview of regenerative therapies

Form of therapy	Status	Field of application	Main advantages	Limitations
Stem cell therapy	Clinically applied, partly experimental	Early to middle stage of osteoarthritis	Regeneration of cartilage tissue, inhibition of inflammation	High costs, limited long-term data
Exosomes	Experimental	Early stages, concomitant	Cell-free therapy, low immune reactions	Lack of long-term studies
PRP (Platelet-Rich Plasma)	Clinically established	Early to middle stage	Growth factor release, anti-inflammatory	Effect often temporary
Gene modulation (CRISPR/Cas9)	Preclinical studies	Future prospects	Potentially causal treatment	Ethical and safety issues

18 Table 4: Influence of psychosocial factors on the course of the disease

Factor	Influence on osteoarthritis	Therapeutic approach
Stress	Increases pain perception, intensifies inflammation	Stress management, relaxation techniques
Depression	Negative influence on motivation, intensification of pain	Cognitive behavioural therapy, ACT
Fear	Promotes avoidance of exercise, chronification	Anxiety reduction through education, exposure
Social isolation	Reduces activity, worsens quality of life	Social integration, group therapy

19 Table 5: Comparison of physical therapy forms

Form of therapy	Effect	Field of application	Evidence base
Heat therapy	Muscle relaxation, pain relief	Chronic osteoarthritis pain	Well documented
Cold therapy	Anti-inflammatory, pain-relieving	Acute relapses, joint effusions	Well documented
TENS	Pain modulation	Chronic pain	Moderately occupied
Magnetic field therapy	Promotes blood circulation, relieves pain	Early stages, complementary therapy	Inconsistent results
Shock wave therapy	Tissue regeneration, pain relief	Early to middle stage	Positive short-term effects

20 Table 6: Overview of drug therapy options for osteoarthritis

Drug group	Examples of active ingredients	Mechanism of action	Advantages	Disadvantages/side effects
Non-steroidal anti-inflammatory drugs (NSAR)	Ibuprofen, Diclofenac, Naproxen	Inhibition of COX enzymes, anti-inflammatory	Rapid pain relief	Gastrointestinal bleeding, kidney dysfunction
COX-2 inhibitors	Celecoxib, etoricoxib	Selective COX-2 inhibition	Lower risk of stomach problems	Increased cardiovascular risk
Corticosteroids (intra-articular)	Triamcinolone, methylprednisolone	Strong anti-inflammatory effect	Effective for acute relapses	Only effective in the short term, cartilage damage with long-term use
Opioids	Tramadol, Tilidine	Central pain inhibition	Can be used in the short term for severe pain	Risk of dependence, sedation
Symptom-modifying drugs (SYSADOAs)	Glucosamine, chondroitin	Supports cartilage metabolism	Well tolerated, long-term effect	Effect scientifically controversial
Biologics	Adalimumab, etanercept	Inhibition of pro-	Reduction of systemic	High costs, risk of infection

Drug group	Examples of active ingredients	Mechanism of action	Advantages	Disadvantages/side effects
		inflammatory cytokines	inflammatory processes	

21 Table 7: Current clinical studies on innovative osteoarthritis therapies (selection)

Study name	Therapeutic approach	Phase	Target population	Main objective
STAR-KNEE	Mesenchymal stem cells	Phase III	Knee osteoarthritis, grade II-III	Cartilage regeneration, pain relief
GENOA	CRISPR/Cas9 based gene modification	Preclinical	Early stage osteoarthritis	Inhibition of MMP-13, promotion of cartilage growth
REPAIR	Exosome therapy	Phase II	Knee and hip arthrosis	Inflammation inhibition, functional improvement
PRIMA	PRP (Platelet-Rich Plasma)	Phase III	Early stage osteoarthritis	Delaying the course of the disease
BIOKART	Combination of stem cells and growth factors	Phase I/II	Cartilage damage after trauma	Improvement of joint function, regeneration of hyaline cartilage

22 Table 8: Prognostic factors for successful treatment of osteoarthritis

Factor	Influence on the success of therapy	Optimisation measure
Stage of the disease	Early stage favourable, late stage complicates treatment success	Early diagnosis and intervention
Body weight	High load with overweight	Weight reduction, change of diet
Muscle function	Well-trained muscles improve joint stability	Physiotherapy, targeted muscle training
Psychosocial factors	Depression and anxiety worsen pain tolerance	Psychotherapeutic support
Therapy compliance	High compliance improves therapy success	Educational measures, self-management

22 Table 9: Summary of the most common biomarkers in osteoarthritis therapy

Biomarkers	Meaning	Clinical application
CRP (C-reactive protein)	Inflammation markers	Assessment of systemic inflammation
CTX-II	Cartilage degradation product	Early detection of cartilage degradation
COMP (Cartilage Oligomeric Matrix Protein)	Cartilage metabolism	Progress monitoring, prognosis assessment
IL-6	Proinflammatory cytokine	Inflammatory activity in the joint
MMP-13	Matrix metalloproteinase, cartilage degradation	Potential therapy target, progression marker

23 Table 10: Preventive measures to avoid and delay osteoarthritis

Measure	Effect	Implementation recommendation
Normalise body weight	Reduces joint stress and inflammatory activity	Balanced diet, regular exercise
Joint-friendly sport	Improving joint stability, maintaining mobility	Swimming, cycling, Nordic walking
Avoidance of overloading	Reduces mechanical microtrauma in the cartilage	Ergonomic working, avoidance of extreme sports
Healthy nutrition	Anti-inflammatory, supports cartilage	Mediterranean diet, omega-3-rich food, antioxidants
Correction of muscular imbalances	Reduces incorrect loading of the joints	Targeted muscle training under physiotherapeutic guidance
Avoidance of risk factors	Reduces systemic inflammation	Stop smoking, stress management, moderate alcohol consumption

24 Table 11: Treatment recommendations according to stage of osteoarthritis

Stage of the disease	Preferred therapy options	Supplementary measures
Early stage (grade I-II)	Lifestyle modification, physical therapy, micronutrient supplementation	PRP injections, initial drug therapy if required
Intermediate stage (grade II-III)	Multimodal therapy, drug-based pain therapy, regenerative procedures (stem cells, exosomes)	Physiotherapy, psychotherapy for pain chronification
Late stage (grade III-IV)	Surgical measures (endoprosthetics), pain therapy	Post-operative rehabilitation, provision of aids

25 Table 12: Overview of innovative therapeutic procedures, success rates and evidence levels

Form of therapy	Success rate (clinical studies)	Evidence level (according to OCEBM*)	Main area of application	Remarks
Stem cell therapy (MSC)	60-80 % subjective improvement	Grade II-III	Early to middle stage of osteoarthritis	Good pain relief, limited long-term data
Exosome therapy	50-70 % improvement	Grade III (experimental)	Early stage, regenerative support	Currently mainly in studies, long-term effect unclear
PRP (Platelet-Rich Plasma)	50-75 % symptomatic improvement	Grade II	Early to middle stage of osteoarthritis	Short-term effect well documented, effect levels off after 6-12 months
CRISPR/Cas9 gene modification	Preclinical, success in animal experiments	Grade V	Future prospects	No clinical authorisation yet, ethical discussions
Low-level laser therapy (LLLT)	40-60 % pain reduction	Grade II-III	Chronic pain conditions	Good results with regular use

Form therapy	Success of rate (clinical studies)	Evidence level (according to OCEBM*)	Main area of application	Remarks
Magnetic field therapy (PEMF)	30-50 % subjective improvement	Grade III	Supplementary measure	Inconsistent study situation, varying individual effectiveness
Shock wave therapy (ESWT)	60-70 % short-term pain relief	Grade II	Early to middle stage	Good short-term success, limited long-term effect

* OCEBM: Oxford Centre for Evidence-Based Medicine - Evidence level I: High-quality randomised trials; level II: Well-designed cohort or case-control studies; level III: Observational studies, level IV: Expert opinion, level V: Theoretical foundations without clinical data.

26 Complete bibliography

1. general principles of osteoarthritis

- Arden, N., & Nevitt, M. C. (2006). Osteoarthritis: Epidemiology. *Best Practice & Research Clinical Rheumatology*, 20(1), 3-25.
  https://doi.org/10.1016/j.berh.2005.09.007

- Felson, D. T. (2010). Osteoarthritis as a disease of mechanics. *Osteoarthritis and Cartilage*, 18(3), 305-310.
  https://doi.org/10.1016/j.joca.2009.12.008

- Hunter, D. J., & Bierma-Zeinstra, S. (2019). Osteoarthritis. *The Lancet*, 393(10182), 1745-1759.
  https://doi.org/10.1016/S0140-6736(19)30417-9

2. classical drug therapy

- Bannuru, R. R., Osani, M. C., Vaysbrot, E. E., et al. (2019). OARSI guidelines for the non-surgical management of knee, hip, and polyarticular osteoarthritis. *Osteoarthritis and Cartilage*, 27(11), 1578-1589.
  https://doi.org/10.1016/j.joca.2019.06.011

- Shapiro, B. H., & Principe, M. F. (2015). The role of dietary supplements in osteoarthritis: Current evidence and recommendations. *Journal of Clinical Rheumatology*, 21(8), 451-457.
  https://doi.org/10.1097/RHU.0000000000000304

3. physical and apparative therapy

- Brosseau, L., Wells, G. A., Brosseau, M., et al. (2012). Low level laser therapy (Classes I, II and III) for treating osteoarthritis. *Cochrane Database of Systematic Reviews*, (12), CD010035. https://doi.org/10.1002/14651858.CD010035

- Zeng, C., Li, H., Yang, T., et al. (2015). Effectiveness of extracorporeal shockwave therapy for knee osteoarthritis: A systematic review and meta-analysis. *Journal of Orthopaedic Research*, 33(5), 659-666. https://doi.org/10.1002/jor.22816

4. nutritional and micronutrient therapy

- Baker, K. R., Matthan, N. R., Lichtenstein, A. H., et al. (2011). Association of plasma phospholipid n-3 and n-6 fatty acids with physical function in mobility-limited older adults. *European Journal of Clinical Nutrition*, 65(3), 282-289. https://doi.org/10.1038/ejcn.2010.261

- Henrotin, Y., Lambert, C., Couchourel, D., Ripoll, C., & Chiotelli, E. (2011). Nutraceuticals: Do they represent a new era in the management of osteoarthritis? *Osteoarthritis and Cartilage*, 19(1), 1-21. https://doi.org/10.1016/j.joca.2010.10.017

5. regenerative and biological therapy approaches

- Barry, F., & Murphy, M. (2013). Mesenchymal stem cells in joint disease and repair. *Nature Reviews Rheumatology*, 9(10), 584-594. https://doi.org/10.1038/nrrheum.2013.109

- Evans, C. H., Ghivizzani, S. C., & Robbins, P. D. (2011). Gene transfer to human joints: Progress toward a gene therapy of arthritis. *PNAS*, 108(48), 19072-19077. https://doi.org/10.1073/pnas.1108293108

- Mendelsohn, A. R., & Larrick, J. W. (2017). CRISPR-Cas9 genome editing for therapeutic applications: Progress and challenges. *Current Molecular Medicine*, 17(2), 98-114. https://doi.org/10.2174/1566524017666170123105211

6. psychological and behavioural therapies

- Kabat-Zinn, J. (1990). *Full Catastrophe Living: Using the Wisdom of Your Body and Mind to Face Stress, Pain, and Illness.* New York: Delacorte.

- McCracken, L. M., & Vowles, K. E. (2014). Acceptance and commitment therapy and mindfulness for chronic pain: Model, process, and progress. *American Psychologist*, 69(2), 178-187. https://doi.org/10.1037/a0035623

- Turk, D. C., & Okifuji, A. (2010). Psychological factors in chronic pain: Evolution and revolution. *Journal of Consulting and Clinical Psychology*, 70(3), 678-690. https://doi.org/10.1037/0022-006X.70.3.678

7. interdisciplinary and multimodal therapy

- Dagenais, S., Caro, J., & Haldeman, S. (2008). A systematic review of low back pain cost of illness studies. *Spine Journal*, 8(1), 8-20. https://doi.org/10.1016/j.spinee.2007.10.005
- Karjalainen, K., Malmivaara, A., van Tulder, M., et al. (2001). Multidisciplinary biopsychosocial rehabilitation for subacute low back pain in working-age adults. *Cochrane Database of Systematic Reviews*, (2), CD002193. https://doi.org/10.1002/14651858.CD002193

8 Personalised medicine and genetic therapy

- Kim, Y. S., Smoak, M. M., Melchiorri, A. J., & Mikos, A. G. (2020). Gene delivery for osteoarthritis therapy. *Journal of Controlled Release*, 317, 285-300. https://doi.org/10.1016/j.jconrel.2019.11.010
- Zeggini, E., Panoutsopoulou, K., Southam, L., et al. (2012). Identification of new susceptibility loci for osteoarthritis: A genome-wide association study. *The*

Lancet, 380(9844), 815-823. https://doi.org/10.1016/S0140-6736(12)60681-3